I0039213

GO!

GO!

One Man's Guide to Health, Vitality and Fat Loss

Ian Tudor

Copyright © 2017 Ian Tudor
Print Edition

All rights reserved. No part of this publication may be reproduced, distributed, or transmitted in any form or by any means, including photocopying, recording, or other electronic or mechanical methods, without the prior written permission of the publisher, except in the case of brief quotations embodied in critical reviews and certain other noncommercial uses permitted by copyright law.

Contents

Introduction

THIS BESTSELLER BOOK YOU ARE about to read puts the power in *your* hands for looking good, feeling great and achieving the body weight most ideal to you.

It is a book on health and vitality offering the most effective methods for performing cardio to obtain optimal fat loss. Combining knowledge gleaned from personal experience, life coaching and research, everything stored within these pages is tried and tested and works regardless of who you are and whatever the level of health, fitness and weight you start at.

If you feel bad about how you look, this book will get you looking good. If you want to experience fat loss but have no idea how to go about it, you will be shown cardio exercises that work and keep on working even when the fat you carry with you right now, is a distant memory.

Depressed, downtrodden, confused, bewildered, unable to quit the binge eating at night, overweight and undervalued? This book will give you a clearly laid out path for reinvigorating your health, for strengthening your mind and for vanquishing your fears and doubts so that you can experience the best life imaginable… in the shortest time frame possible.

Everything you need to know about health, vitality

and fat loss is told here from setting your goals and learning about yourself to understanding what to eat and why and following the personal stories of those who have achieved success.

In every chapter there are top tips that will save you time and effort enabling you to accelerate towards your desired destination.

Nothing and no one can hold you back from achieving your goal.

Let this be the beginning of your fat loss journey and the end.

Transform yourself, transform your life – the power to achieve this rests is in your hands.

CHAPTER ONE

Your Goal

"Nothing can stop the man with the right mental attitude from achieving his goal, nothing on earth can help the man with the wrong mental attitude"
Thomas Jefferson

TO ACHIEVE ANYTHING GOOD IN life the right mental attitude is crucial. It is the governing factor behind whether you reach your goal or you do *not* reach your goal. Great men, like Jefferson, know intrinsically that a person's inner being always manifests itself outwards. By this we mean that whatever is contained within the individual, good or bad, will always impact upon their actions.

By examining, therefore whom we are inside and making the relevant adjustments before we embark on a journey or a goal is both prudent and necessary.

We will discuss *'Cultivating the Right Mental Attitude'* in Chapter Three, for now simply raising the awareness that **attitude is fundamental to success** will suffice.

The Importance of a Goal

In any arena of life having a goal is key to finding a sense of purpose and meaning to our actions. It gives us a satisfaction that we are progressing as well as improving who we are. Both these combined make us feel alive and good about ourselves, confident that we are living our lives to the full and not merely existing.

A goal gives us something to measure ourselves by. Without fixed point in the distance to aim for, we are the human equivalent of leaves blowing in the wind, swept in any which direction and arriving neither here nor there.

Setting A Goal

In setting a goal you need to:

i. Create your desire: In this case, your ideal bodyweight. This needs to be within the boundaries of good health.

ii. Choose a fixed date in the future for when your ideal bodyweight will be achieved, make it realistic and stick to it. The fixing of a specific date is a powerful mental marker that when focused is a motivating force. It enables you to work day-by-day, week-by-week achievements.

Let's say for example, you are 250 pounds and your bodyweight goal is 195 pounds. You have given yourself 12 weeks in order to lose this weight. This means that you will need to lose around four-five pounds per week. Having a measurable target makes this goal much easier to achieve.

iii. Set a bodyweight goal that scares you. Something that

seems impossible. Be totally unreasonable in setting the bar high, perhaps to the weight you were when you left school or first met your partner.

Or set the bar higher than it has ever been before, (*go on, you can do it*) keeping always wisely within the boundaries of good health.

Remember the goal needs to be *your* goal, not someone else's goal for you.

iv. Visualization: The imaging faculty of the human mind is incredibly powerful more so than any telescope or microscope. It is our immense capacity for imagination that sets us apart from all other living creatures.

Imagining or visualizing what we want and holding the image in our minds with the expectancy that what we seek will be found is a concept that is recognized widely in spiritual writings. It is a powerful almost holy tool humans possess that provides them with an unrivalled form of creative freedom.

In order to activate the law of attraction, you must see in your mind's eye the very thing you desire, as already achieved.

Go on try it. Take a peak at yourself 84 pounds lighter. Look at those curves, see how those trousers hang off your waist – a waist, look you have a waist. Imagine the compliments you will get and the respect for all your efforts. Imagine your sense of self worth.

Try seeing this image over and over again as frequently as possible adding more layers of detail and clarity with each passing day until you reach a state of maximum mental clarity.

Wow, this is me, I look great.

By shifting your conscious mind back and forth on the subject of your weight loss you will be giving your brain something it can 'hunt down'.

The mental exercise of visualizing can be done at any time of the day or night, whenever your mind has some 'downtime'. Once you have your brain in 'hunting' mode, it will be doing everything it can to create a positive outcome on your behalf. It has a focus therefore *you* have a focus.

Imagine, the new you.

Within a matter of days, you will find that circumstances/events/people are all working in your favor, causing a cascade of positive effects.

Be prepared for miracles.

This new super improved vision of your future self is your blue print for success. Keep it in mind at all times when undertaking the upcoming steps throughout this book.

Let nothing or no one obscure the vision you have created.

Keep the image crystal clear and it will empower you to keep on going.

Driving The Goal Into The Mind

Ever wondered why advertisers feel the need to repeat their adverts every TV break? Or enforce what they are saying over and over again?

And in the process spend millions on ad campaigns?

The reason: because adverts influence people to take

action. Fact.

Repeating something over and over again has the effect of driving the message home.

If advertisers can do it, so can we. We have a goal. We have a fixed date by which we need to achieve that goal. We know what that goal is, we can see, touch, taste, smell the goal in our mind's eye.

Now we know what our goal is and can see it, we need to start influencing our brains to take action.

Understanding the advertising industry's method of repetition and frequency of exposure enables us to adopt the same method for our own personal advancement.

Repeating the goal to ourselves over and over again at key times during the day and night ideally upon waking and going to sleep, times when the mind is most susceptible to influence, will kick start the brain into action.

Method

Upon rising in the morning, write out your weight loss goal including the date of completion, 10 times.

In order to have the maximum impact on the mind the goal must be written out as being already achieved, as this registers in the present tense and your subconscious can only process present tense, positive affirmation statements.

And always start with the pronoun 'I'. *You* are the only person in the universe qualified to use the word 'I'.

To understand the power of writing out your goal, try visualizing the sub conscious as an office worker receiving a command from Head Office. 'I am 210 pounds is the command and the subconscious sets to work making the 210 pounds a reality.

1. I am 210 pounds today July 15th!
2. I am 210 pounds, today July 15th!
3. I am 210 pounds today July 15th!
5. I am 210 pounds today July 15th!
6. I am 210 pounds today July 15th!
7. I am 210 pounds today July 15th!
8. I am 210 pounds today July 15th!
9. I am 210 pounds today July 15th!
10. I am 210 pounds today July 15th!

Make writing this out the first thing you do when you wake up.

Repeat this ritual before going to bed. Make it your last activity before sleep. Performing this ritual before falling asleep at night is when it is most effectual. As you drift into sleep, the goal will pass into your subconscious mind, which in a state of rest has time to start putting your goal into action. You will wake up with the insights and solutions that will further you towards your goal.

The simple straightforward practice of writing out your goal both in the morning and at night has been proven time and again to have highly positive psychological effects that can only be understood and fully appreciated by the person undertaking the experience in other words, You.

You become your own advertising agency only instead of being told what action to take you are initiating the action, in control of your own psychological reins. This makes the effect all the more powerful as it is something *you* wholeheartedly desire.

After seven days of writing out your goals ten times morning and night, you can speak out loud your goal a further ten times to really get your message across.

It is vitally important that when you speak out loud your goal statement you emotionalize it. Insert energy and purpose into your words. Incredibly, the subconscious mind processes emotive statements far more effectively than those spoken in bland monotones.

Exposing the mind twice a day to your desired goal will supercharge your efforts and cause you to move with a sense of urgency in regard to achieving your goal. This practice and simple discipline lies at the foundation of success and like all motivational steps, requires diligence.

It is, however, as important if not more so than the exercise and nutritional components outlined later in the book.

Be prepared to experience the arrival of brilliance into your life by making your desired goal the focus of your infinitely powerful mind.

Top Tip

Remember this is *your* goal. It belongs to no one else but *you*.

At this stage in your journey, you might feel inclined to share your goal with someone else. Resist from doing this. When you put your goal out in the world, you are compromising the great driving force contained within it, dampening down the flickering spark of desire.

In addition, you are putting your goal, dreams and desires at the mercy of everyone else's scrutiny. With scrutiny come negative perceptions and judgments often from individuals who feel the need for whatever reason, normally because of their own lack of self worth, to assign their selves the role of moral/practical coach or weight loss guru.

On questioning these supposedly 'helpful' individuals you will find they generally lack any goals of their own thus will take immense pleasure out of sucking the lifeblood from yours. Don't go there. This is *your* goal keep it private and focus on growing that flickering spark into a blazing flame.

Recap:

Set a Goal.

Create your own desired bodyweight – yours and yours alone.

Fix a date for when your goal will be achieved.

Visualize your goal at all times.

Write your achieved goal out ten times morning and night.

Keep your goal private.

Case Study

*"The danger lies not in setting your goal too high
and missing it but in setting it too low and
hitting it"*
Michelangelo

David's Story

David was 365 pounds and had been for the past seven years. A 28 year old factory supervisor he had tried half a dozen or more times to reduce his bodyweight using different diet and training regimes at several local gyms.

To begin, there was always great success, the loss of 25 – 35 pounds in the first couple of weeks. Pleased with the instant results, David had the tendency to lessen his resolve. What harm from the odd sweet or from skipping a cardio session? Within the identical time it took him to lose the weight, it returned. He was back to 365 pounds, depressed and full of self-loathing that his supportive spouse, Sharon should see him fail again.

Tired from carrying all the extra weight, despondent and fed up he would arrive home from work and slump onto the sofa putting his arm around his beloved Sharon, ready to watch TV, as normal. Over the last decade since getting together, Sharon had always been there for David in all his various shapes and sizes.

"Never mind, Dave," she would say patting his chubby arm. "There's always next year you can try again then. And you know that I love you all the same. Don't you?"

David would simply sighed in response and settle

down to gaze at the telly, aware that Sharon was only being kind.

Interpretation

David started out with every good intention to lose a significant amount of bodyweight. He was determined and diligent in all the essential areas of diet and training. What he lacked though, was a goal. He knew he wanted to lose weight but had no measurable weight loss goal in mind. In addition, he had no fixed date in which his goal could be achieved. His was a wishy-washy regime. He knew he didn't want a 365 pound body but not what he *did* want and *by* when.

This type of guess strategy is always doomed to fail.

Outcome

When David became one of my clients, my first suggestion to him was to set a hugely unreasonable weight loss goal.

"Did you say 225 pounds?" He asked me in disbelief. "It has been almost fifteen years since I was that weight. Could this even be possible?"

Today David is 196 pounds and no longer works as a factory supervisor. His increased confidence from smashing through his goal inspired him to look for a new career. He works now in investment banking. Last year he and Sharon had a white wedding and David was every bit the dashing groom.

CHAPTER TWO

Your Cardio Program to Shedding Pounds

*"First you start by doing what is possible and
before long you are doing the impossible"*
St Francis of Assisi

ALL GREAT AND BRILLIANT ACCOMPLISHMENTS BEGIN with taking a few small steps at a time, doing what is within your capabilities when you start out and using that perfect blend of consistency with perseverance. Keep going and within a week or so, you will have made measurable progress.

This applies to learning any skill, from musical instruments to riding a bike but when it comes to health, fitness and losing weight, the results are almost instantaneous.

Why?

Because your body *wants* you to succeed, it *wants* you to get fitter, slimmer and healthier and is sending positive signals of encouragement every step of the way. After just a few weeks you will look back at your starting point and see/feel instantly how far you have come.

This chapter is all about cardiovascular exercise. How the proper application of cardio is the foundation of health, wellbeing and fat loss.

Optimum Time for Burning Fat

Wake Up and Go

While asleep, the body uses calories to maintain energy to the vital functions such as the heart, lungs and brain along with a plethora of other processes also requiring energy to function.

Over night, your body will have been placed into a calorie deficit meaning any cardio performed on waking up will dip directly into your fat stores as an alternate source of energy.

You exercise, you burn up fat. What joy. Not only have you woken to see another day you have also reduced a considerable number of fat cells before your digestive system has even kicked into action.

Do this every morning for a few mornings and very quickly that clever body of yours, (your number one fan) will be getting into the whole pre-breakfast-cardio-exercising-routine ordering the liver to release energy in the form of glycogen directly to your muscles. This will enable you to perform your exercises with full vigor and verve thus optimizing your workout to ensure maximum fat reduction.

Optimum Duration for Maximum Fat Burn

10 Minutes A Day

Get away, 10 minutes? Is that all?
　　Yep. That's all.

More is (Not) Better

When we perform any form of physical exercise it

constitutes a stress imposed on the body. This stress varies according to the type of exercise as well as other factors namely the duration of exercise and its intensity.

By adopting a 'More is Better' approach to exercise you will be working directly against your Goal of sustained fat reduction as well as damaging your health. One, two, three hours of intense exercise and marathon workout sessions will not shed your pounds. If anything, you will increase in weight.

Intense exercise = increased calories

Intense exercise = increased stress on body = increased risk of permanent damage to the body.

So, 10 minutes. That's all it takes. 10 minutes daily when you wake up so long, as you combine these exercises with the correct fat burning diet coming up in the *Nutrition* chapter.

Six Benefits of Cardiovascular Exercise on Everyday Life

1. It reduces blood pressure, which in turn reduces stress

2. It elevates the mood, which helps to eliminate depression by causing the release of neurotransmitters known as endorphins, which are responsible for blocking pain and enhancing positive emotion.

3. It increases your blood circulation by 40% and your brain function by 60%. This means better concentration and improved memory.

4. It significantly reduces your risk of cancer and

osteoporosis, prevents heart problems and lessens the likelihood of strokes.

5. It aids with the digestion of foods and nutrients

6. It boosts your immune system.

The Benefits of Losing Weight

In addition to the above six benefits, which are part and parcel of a happy, healthy You, cardiovascular exercise elevates the metabolism and keeps the body burning fat when you are both awake and asleep.

Before looking at this in more details let us first of all grapple with some of the common misconceptions when it comes to cardiovascular exercising.

No Pain No Gain?

Makes perfect sense yes? We have all seen the movie where the protagonist in an attempt to outrival his archenemy, strides into a gym and undertakes a grueling workout causing his veins to bulge all the while spurred on by a mentor, *"You can do it, Jimmy."* Or from the sidelines by us the viewer caught up in the thrill of an adrenalin-fuelled heavy rock soundtrack.

'More is Better', 'No Pain No Gain'

Well, sorry folks but that is just movie-speak.

In reality:

'More is better' = increased stress on your central nervous system causing the body to slow down internally and hold on to body fat

'No pain no gain' = equals increased stress on your

central nervous system causing the body to slow down internally and hold on to body fat.

From this approach expect only disappointment, injury and zero results.

Here is why.

Cardio workouts exert a stress on the heart and lungs and on the liver, which is considered the engine of the body as it releases glycogen, the raw energy needed to undertake cardiovascular or indeed any exercise. Forcing the body to endure more and more cardio for longer periods increases the overall stress on the body's central nervous system.

This, in turn, leads to a higher demand for calories, as the liver has to work harder to release glycogen, which comes from the energy in food.

So, what happens next? You work out three hours and you feel a million dollars. How have you managed to work out three hours? By matching your exercise with calories.

Outcome: Your weight has stayed the same or in some cases, increased.

So, what do we do?

We work out harder and we balance this with eating more calories – remember, your body knows best. Of course, we try to reduce the calories but in doing so, we reduce our energy levels for working out.

In the end we fail. It must be bad genetics. Right?

Wrong!

You can burn fat through cardiovascular exercising efficiently, safely and effectively, if you follow this method.

Method

In order to burn fat through cardiovascular exercising you need to get up close and personal with your body.

Being in touch with how your body functions physiologically is essential to your success. Your body is your best friend. The kindest thing you can do for yourself is to listen to it and learn from it.

Your Cardiovascular Exercise Toolkit

These exercises if undertaken *at the right time of day*, for the *correct duration* in combination with a *fat burning diet*, ensure you shed pounds.

They are listed in a hierarchical form. The most important exercises, namely those that incorporate the larger muscles and are likely to lead to the most breathlessness, are listed first.

All these exercises are to be undertaken from a **standing position** on a level floor surface:

1. The Partial Squat

The *Partial Squat* is one of the many versions of squat, which come under the umbrella term, 'King of Exercise'. A strong squat means a strong body.

The first reference to the idea of the squat as an exercise form was in a book written by strongman, Eugene Sandow, the world's first official weightlifter and the inspiration for the Sandow Trophy given annually to the winner of the Mr Olympia title. Sandow was revered not only for his strength but also for his physique, which he attributed to regular squatting exercises.

The *Partial Squat* is an excellent starting movement to

use, as it will get the heart rate up in just a few repetitions. This exercise provides low impact on the knees as it ensures solid stability from both legs.

To perform the *Partial Squat,* stand upright with feet a little over shoulder width apart. Ensure your feet are pointing in a ten-to-two clock face position in order to allow the knees to move in a natural range of motion.

Once the position is assumed, cross the arms at the wrists in front of the chest and lift your chin a little, focusing your eyes on a fixed point ahead such as a curtain rail. Fixing your gaze before you begin will allow for best posture.

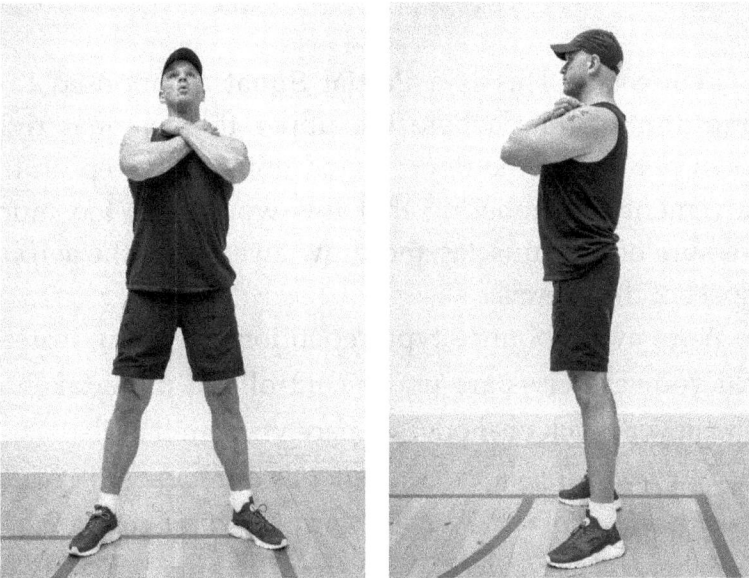

Bend your knees whilst breathing in. Hold your breath. Return to the starting position and exhale. Repeat this movement over and again.

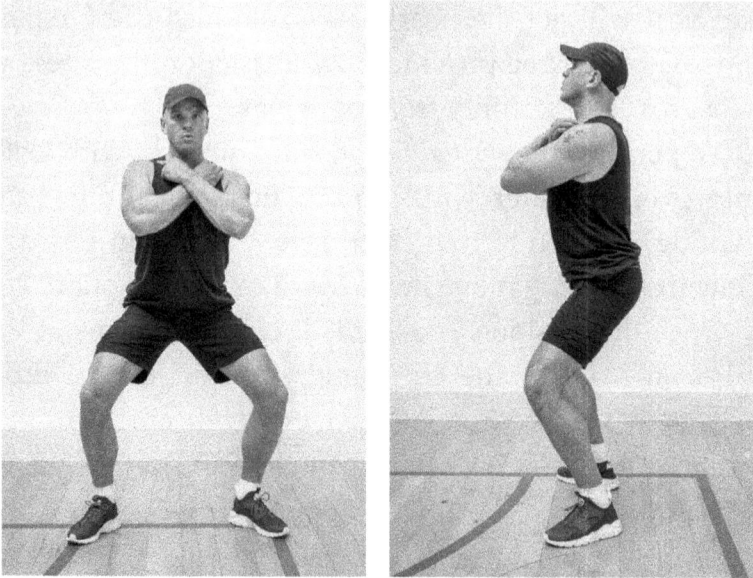

Remember: This is a **Partial Squat** as opposed to a **Traditional Squat** where the upper thighs squat right down parallel to the floor. Avoid going too deep on the movement remembering that this would put too much pressure on the muscles and draw away from the aerobic aspect of the exercise.

Also, avoid bounce type repetitions ensuring instead that your exercises are under control and undertaken at whichever quick or moderate pace you can handle.

*Take heart: If you perform only this **one** exercise in combination with a **correct diet**, it would suffice in you losing as much body fat as required.*

2. The Air Punch Drill

The *Air Punch Drill* is FUN and can be as moderate or vigorous as you wish it to be. It is not a complicated exercise in that it feels natural. It can, as with any of these exercises, be performed by you deciding on a set amount of repetitions you wish to achieve or by you challenging your time against the clock.

To perform the *Air Punch Drill*, stand on the spot and raise your arms up in front of you, sleepwalking style. This is the most natural position to hold out the arms and hands.

Close both hands into fists with a moderate but not too tense grip. Establish which hand is your primary lead punch hand, in other words which hand you would naturally favor in throwing your first punch, left or right. If the right is the natural punching hand then also take a right step forward and slightly bend at the knees to give you your natural boxers stance. If the left hand is your primary punch hand then do exactly the same stance except stepping forward with the left leg, again with a slight bend in the knees. Tuck your chin in and tilt your forehead forwards. This stance is called the *Boxer's Crouch*.

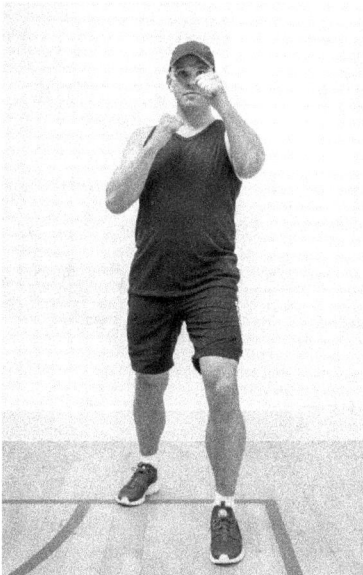

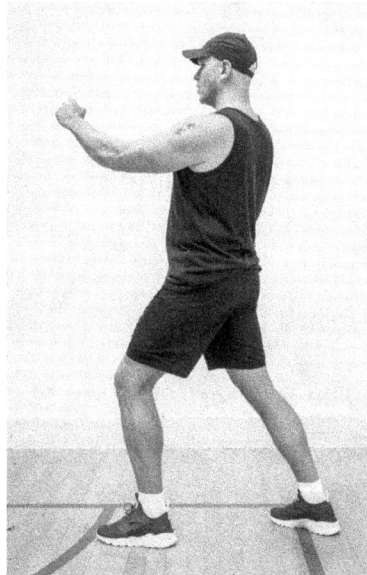

From this position, throw your lead punch quickly followed by your secondary punch and repeat the movement.

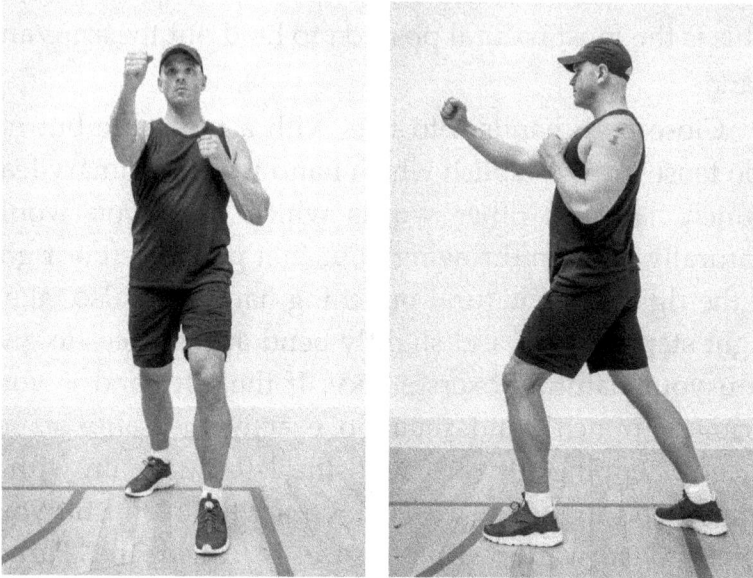

Avoid over extending when you throw each punch and twisting your torso. The punches should be moderate in extension and as quick as possible within a moderate pace.

Speed and fluidity of movement are key elements of this exercise and these are facilitated by the use of proper balance. Maintain a slight bend in the knees and keep the forward footstep of the lead hand as aforementioned.

3. The Supported Muay Thai Knee

The *Supported Muay Thai Knee* dates back to the 16th Century when the famous Siamese fighter, Nai Khanomtom invented it as a means of fighting for his freedom from the Burmese. It was introduced into British boxing in 1913.

In terms of our exercises, it promotes good balance and posture.

To perform the *Supported Muay Thai Knee*, stand facing a wall and place both hands on the wall, slightly wider than shoulder width apart and raised a little above shoulder height.

Lean forward into the wall ensuring your feet are shoulder width apart positioned behind your hips in a diagonal stance, leaning forward into the wall.

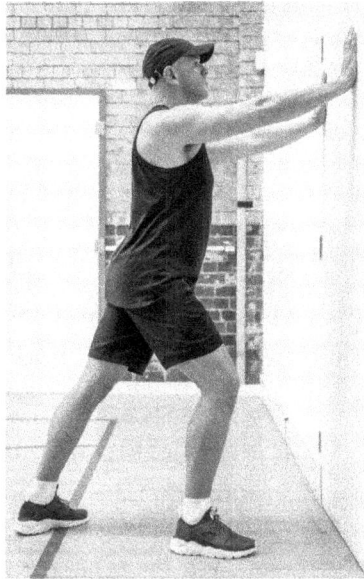

Maintaining this forward leaning position, lift one knee up to approximately 90 degrees from your torso and back down again. Repeat the exercise using the same leg. As you gather a feel for the movement, gradually increase your speed counting the repetitions as you go. A favorable number of repetitions for each leg would be between five and twenty. Once this number has been achieved, move on to the opposing leg.

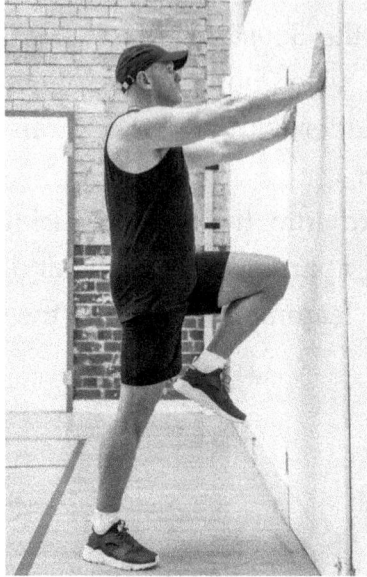

Avoid standing upright as this causes the knee to make contact with the wall. It works best if you accentuate the forward leaning into the wall so as to provide a clear path for the knee to travel.

As you gain confidence performing this exercise, the knee should be thrown with the same fluidity as the arms in an *Air Punch Drill* in a free flowing formation.

4. Supported Uppercut and Hook

The *Supported Uppercut and Hook* is an effective mixed martial arts self defense tool developed originally to enable combatants to strike in the clinch phase of a fight. The word, 'clinch', referring to when two fighters are locked together in a standing position.

To perform the *Supported Uppercut and Hook*, stand facing the wall placing both hands on the wall shoulder width apart. With your feet slightly wider than shoulder width apart, lean forward into the wall. Keeping one hand on the wall for support, take your opposing hand and throw an *Uppercut*. This means keeping your arm bent and delivering a punch in an upward motion.

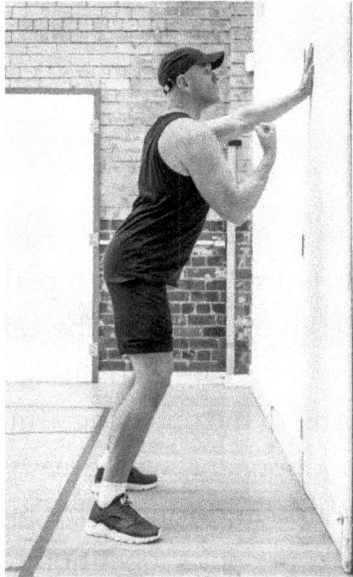

Repeat the movement, a repetition range of between 10 and 20 is a good starting point that you can increase later on.

Maintaining your position and using the same arm, throw the *Hook*. This requires you to lift your fist up from the waist and sweep it across the torso and inward at head level. The path of the punch should resemble the shape of its namesake a *'Hook'*.

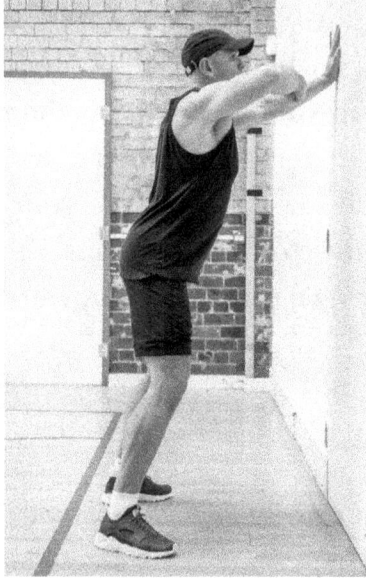

Repeat the movement again at a repetition range of 10 to 20. After this, you can combine the *Uppercut and Hook* in a manner that suits you, counting the repetitions before alternating on to the opposing arm.

Imagining an opponent will greatly increase your levels of motivation in performing this movement as will attempting to beat a previous repetition range.

5. The Clean and Press Without Resistance

The *Clean and Press Without Resistance* originates from weightlifting where athletes attempt to pick up a weighted Olympic bar from the floor and in a singular movement, swing the bar up to shoulder level and raise it overhead using momentum and force from the legs, shoulders and arms.

This movement is fantastic because it involves the lower and upper body combined within one clean crisp movement.

Our adapted cardio version involves little or no weight at all as our aim is to derive an aerobic benefit in order to burn fat.

To perform the *Clean and Press Without Resistance*, you need an empty bar, pole or broom handle. Grasp the bar or pole in an overhand position slightly wider than shoulder width and widen your stance wider than shoulder width apart.

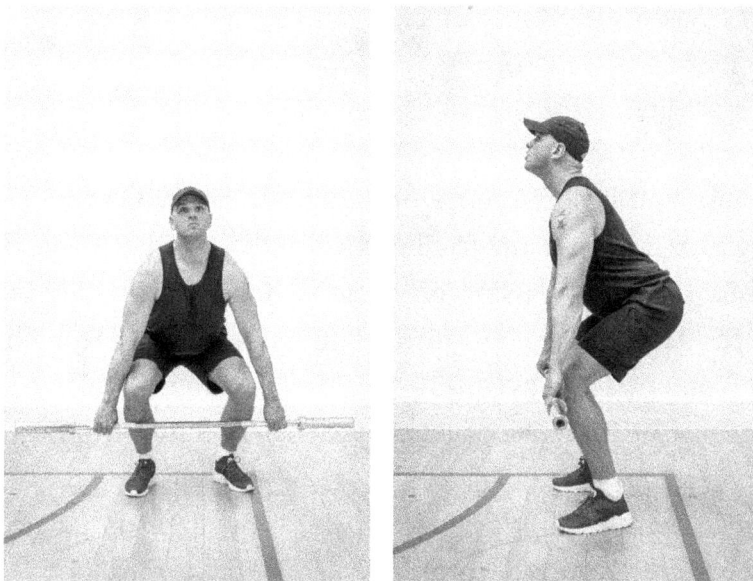

Holding the bar in the overhand position at waist height, bend your knees and keep your chin slightly raised. Ensure the lower back or small of your back is straight to maintain good posture and prevent injury. Now, stand upright and raise the bar to shoulder height and lift overhead in one continuous motion. Repeat this exercise.

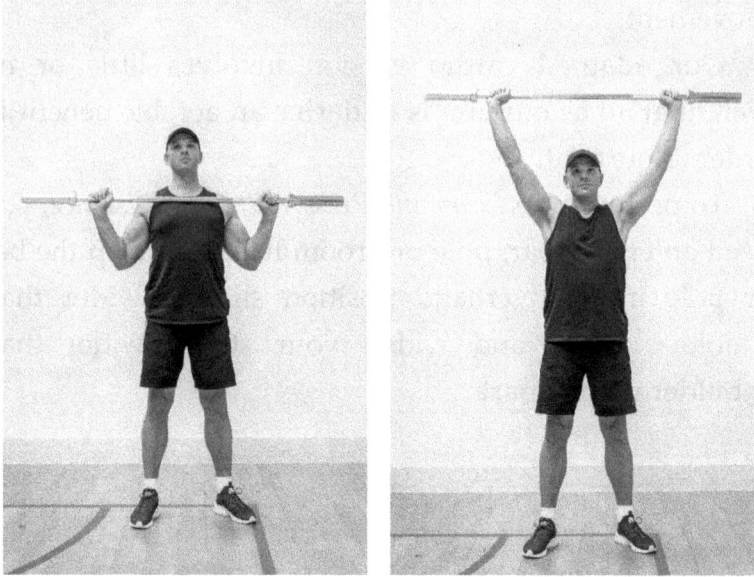

As you become more proficient at this, you may add weights to a bar up to 5kg each side. Alternatively, try dumbbells again using no more than approximately 5kg each dumbbell. The starting repetition range for this movement is between 10 to 20 repetitions, which can always be increased later as you become fitter and stronger.

The dumbbell variation of the movement is particularly effective if a certain side of the upper body is injured, the *Clean and Press Without Resistance* can be performed using a single dumbbell, enabling you to successfully perform a great workout whilst allowing for recovery of any upper body left or right side injury.

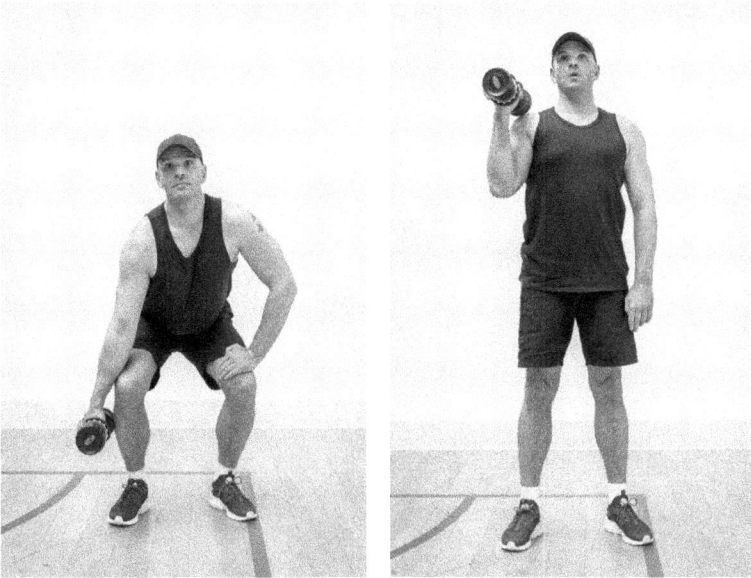

6. Military Press

The *Military Press* is also derived from weightlifting used specifically as a training movement to strengthen shoulders enabling the lifting of heavier weights in the *Clean and Press Without Resistance.*

This movement although less demanding on the cardiovascular system is excellent either as a general warm up movement or for training around a particular injury or imbalance, as it involves no lower body or back movement and can also be performed whilst in a **seated position**.

To perform the *Military Press*, grasp an empty bar or pole in an overhand grip. From the waist position lift or "clean" the bar up to the shoulders maintaining a grip slightly wider than shoulder width.

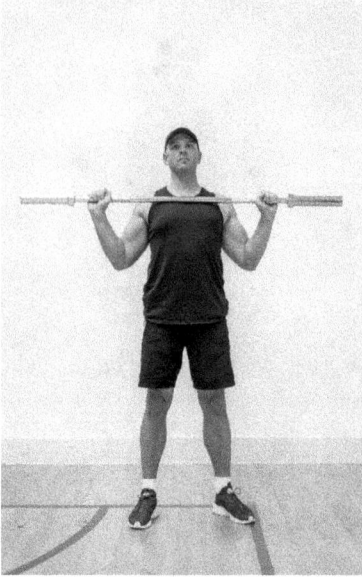

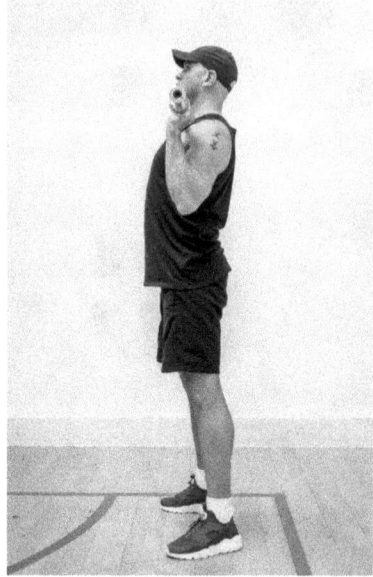

In this position, press the bar up overhead and repeat the movement with a starting repetition range of between 20 to 50 repetitions.

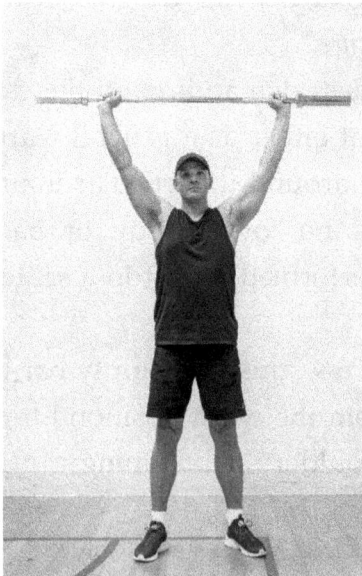

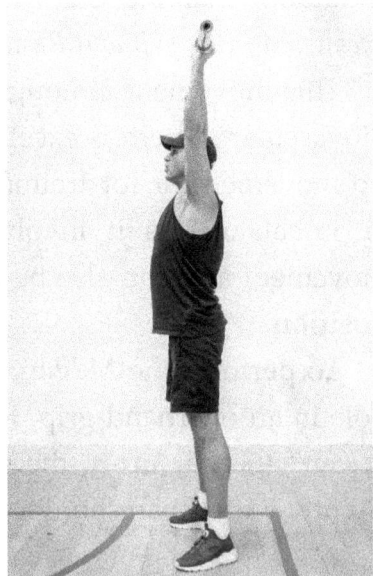

The repetitions should be performed as fast as possible in order to generate maximum benefit to the cardiovascular system.

As you become fitter, weight can be added to a bar although no more than 5kg per side of the bar is recommended, keeping the focus on the cardio aspect of the movement as opposed to turning the movement into a weightlifting exercise.

A variation of the movement can be performed with dumbbells in the same way starting with empty dumbbell handles and slowly increasing the weight of the dumbbells each week exceeding no more than 5kg each side. Again, this dumbbell variation on the exercise can be done using just one dumbbell if a particular side of the body is injured.

7. Step up and Stair Climb

The *Step Up and Stair Climb* is reliably, exactly as it says on the tin. Stepping up on to a fixed platform or surface as well as stair climbing is for many of us, a natural, everyday motion requiring little or no thought.

Stepping and Stair Climbing is hugely beneficial to health. As well as being of benefit to the cardiovascular system, it also develops fitness and confidence that flights of stairs or even several flights of stairs can be climbed with relative ease.

To perform the *Step Up and Stair Climb*, simply find a step or solid platform and step on to it then step back down and repeat the movement with a starting repetition range of between 20 to 50 repetitions. Be mindful of the number of repetitions or write the amount of repetitions down in a simple exercise journal for increasing each time.

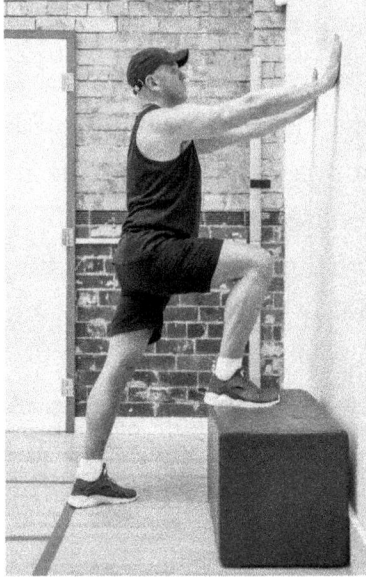

After becoming fitter from increasing the repetitions and losing a significant amount of body fat, you can move onto stair climbing using a flight of steps in or near your home. Again, make a note of the number of consecutive flights you climb and challenge yourself to go one better next time to beat your record.

When starting out on the basic step up movement make use of handrails to hold on to in order to maintain balance as well as safety. Also, you are recommended not to move on to stair climbing until a significant amount of body fat has been shed as it presents a greater impact on the joints. Progress but above all else, use common sense.

The various cardio exercises contained within this book should be looked upon as tools at your disposal. If a particular movement affects an injury or causes discomfort, simply substitute the movement with another more appropriate one.

Four of the Most Common Cardio Mistakes

Performing an Intense Cardiovascular Workout with No Build Up when Overweight

This can impose a significant strain on the heart. The heart is already overworked from the excess weight it has to carry. The dangers of this are heart attack or stroke although this is rare. Another more likely scenario is permanent damage to the heart muscle, which will not necessarily show up without the use of professional medical equipment. There is also the risk of acquiring an injury to joints.

The simple solution to avoiding the above dangers is to start gentle cardio, mindful that you are working *with* the body rather than forcing it to do what it is not accustomed to. Your fitness level will increase providing you start slowly and lose a little more weight, gaining momentum each week.

Cardiovascular Exercising Combined with Poor Nutrition

What you eat will to a large extent govern health, wellbeing and weight.

When an individual consumes a diet of processed highly refined foods, it can be likened to putting diesel fuel into an engine designed to run on petrol. The engine will continue to run but its performance along with power output and longevity will be greatly reduced.

There are some diets touted as 'healthy' that combined with cardiovascular exercises, place an immense burden on the body. Some well known diets such as those which enforce the eating of only low carb foods has been found to be not only unhealthy but also dangerous when combined with exercise.

Eating Breakfast Before Cardio Exercises

We have discussed the whys and wherefores of undertaking cardio exercises before breakfast as the optimum time for shedding pounds. I extol these benefits on a weekly basis to my clients and so am all too often surprised when they inform me that now they have arrived at their ideal body weight, they are postponing exercises until after their bowl of porridge.

"And that is working?" I ask them.

The common reply is, "Well, as I am the weight I want to be, I don't see why the sequence of events matters anymore."

Here, through gritted teeth, I explain that it does matter. In order to maintain a healthy body weight, proper sequencing is crucial.

Of course we all are guilty of having our good intentions slip. I would love to know how many New Year Resolutions still hold by February 1st. That said, maintaining good habits particularly when it comes to remaining slimmed down, is vital for long-term success.

Performing Cardio Involving a joint or other Injury.

If you have a twinge in your knee, a pain in your lower back, a stiff neck you might consider the most obvious way to relieve it is to block book yourself into a series of fitness or training sessions. You might be hoping that through training and working out, you will be able to cure the injury. This however is rarely how it pans out. More than likely, you will attend the classes you have paid for in advance and therefore do not want to skip but in the process, do more harm than good.

In this scenario, there is only one solution and this is to stop. Stop and assess. If necessary, get it checked out. Once you have figured out the nature of the injury, you can act accordingly.

Top Tip

When performing your 10 minutes of cardio, use a beep timer, set to five two-minute intervals. This breaks the cardio down into manageable chunks enabling you to better keep track of the 10-minute time period, as well as enabling you to alternate or change the movement on the sound of each beep.

This simple addition of a beep timer adds a positive dimension to cardio training as psychologically you are only working from one beep to the next as opposed to one long 10-minute period of cardio without any indication of time elapsed. You will find it works better to boost your motivation.

Another enhancement of your cardio is working out to your favorite upbeat tracks in the form of a playlist from a smart phone or other music device. This can supercharge your workouts making you feel fantastic as you take one more step towards achieving your Goal.

Recap:

Cardiovascular exercises when applied properly elevate the metabolism and keep the body burning fat all day.

Best time for cardio exercising is before breakfast.

Ten minutes of exercise is all you need every day.

More exercise is NEVER better.

Intense cardiovascular workout with no build up when overweight leads to risk of heart attacks, strokes, injury to heart muscles or joints.

Seven exercises for daily ten-minute cardio workouts.

For extra motivation, use a beep timer to set your cardiovascular workouts into x five 2-minute intervals.

Case Study

"It does not matter how slow you go so long as
you keep going"
Confucius

Peter's Story

Peter had been overweight for well over a decade and a half. At 47 he had a bodyweight of 266 pounds and was just shy of 5ft 4 inches in height. The weight problem began 17 years before when aged 30, Peter left his former position as a landscape gardener and took a job driving a taxi. Aged 30, Peter's bodyweight was 140 pounds and he had a 28 inch waist, but during his 17 year career as a taxi driver, the long, unsociable shifts had lead him into the habit of eating convenience foods. This combined with a lack of physical activity caused his bodyweight to creep up to 266 pounds an almost 100% increase. Peter had some blood tests that revealed he was on the verge of diabetes combined with high levels of cholesterol in his blood.

Peter's GP was concerned with Peter's poor state of health causing Peter himself to worry.

What particularly upset Peter was not being able to play outdoors or pick up his grandson without becoming breathless due to his additional body fat. Deciding it was time for a change, he remembered the doctor advising that a program of structured exercise could go some way towards reducing his bodyweight whilst contributing towards getting his blood results into a normal range.

Peter was motivated and determined to change.

Pondering his next course of action Peter decided that if years of inactivity had lead him to this level of poor health then surely the solution to regaining health was to an exercise program involving high levels of physical activity; a no brainer by all accounts, as a means to eradicating his health concerns.

The next day he trawled the Internet for an exercise program that met with the criteria of intense physical activity. He found a 12-week military style boot camp with the accompanying description:

'Overweight? Unfit?
Give us 12 weeks to put you through your paces and
get you into the best shape of your life!

Underneath was a pricing list of the various packages on offer as well as a phone number. The 12-week package cost $600 and could be paid in $50 weekly installments. Without hesitation, Peter booked himself a place.

Boot camp began at 6am every day at a *Strength and Conditioning* gym near Peter's house. To get there for 6am, Peter had to swap his shifts from night to day, which was of no concern, as he was determined and prepared to do whatever it took to lose the weight. He owed it to himself and to his family, especially his 9-year old grandson, Ruben.

There was a mixture of overweight shapes and sizes starting boot camp that Monday morning. After filling out an application form including some medical questions, the trainer stood before the group of 15 and explained what the training entailed in terms of exercises as well as a basic weight reducing diet. Today was an induction for the course with the regime getting into full swing the next day.

After the induction talk, Peter began 30 minutes of exercise, which consisted of a light 10-minute slow jog followed by some exercises to get the joints warm in preparation for a 20-minute workout. Peter moved on to the first workout, which was to carry two moderately weighted dumbbells around a circuit of cones. After five minutes performing this particular exercise he moved on to the next and so on and so forth doing five minutes of constant work on each exercise. After 20 minutes, an exhausted Peter had performed four exercises and therefore completed his first workout.

He was very proud of himself, took a shower and went back to his cab to begin his day shift.

That day on the cab he made a concerted effort to follow the nutritional advice handed out by the course, eating meals containing high amounts of protein along with being low in carbohydrate content as according to the trainer, this high protein, low carb approach, would promote fat reduction. Instead of his usual pastry or fry up breakfast Peter opted for a chicken breast with a small salad box and a smaller than usual potato. He felt more optimistic about his future with every mouthful.

The next day he showed up at 6am and began working out at the gym this time for an hour. Once again he felt proud he was moving forward, showered and changed, beginning his day shift on the cab.

All week he showed up at 6am to perform the hour-long grueling physical regime.

After a week of training he had shed 5lbs in body-weight but felt exhausted as well as having picked up some niggling pain in his ankles, knees and hips. He was determined not to quit and took a "No Pain No Gain" attitude towards his situation. 'It will be all worth it in the end', he thought.

After another week he had lost an additional 3lbs in bodyweight but was now exhausted to the point he felt irritable at work. His previously minor niggles were now minor strains. Two weeks in and he was chronically fatigued along with acquiring injuries that would prevent him doing any more exercise for a long while. In short he quit. It was the only option.

Interpretation

Peter had neglected his health for well over a decade not exercising or even moving around a great deal. This sedentary lifestyle combined with eating processed convenience foods led him to gain weight and develop lifestyle related health problems. Peter's logical conclusion was to embark on the extreme opposite of his sedentary lifestyle by implementing a high volume high intensity-training regime.

At the root of Peter's thinking was the widely held assumption that 'More is Better. *If I put in a lot of hours, I will limber up and shed those pounds.'*

With this assumption Peter threw himself with gusto into the new regime. What he didn't realize was that the level of intense physical activity was creating a great amount of stress on his system along with an increased strain on his heart due to his weight.

Unaware that recovery from any type of physical activity is finite, he continued at a dramatic rate, undertaking more workouts thus digging deeper into his limited recoverability. In addition, the sheer volume of exercise led him into chronic fatigue, acquiring minor injuries along the way.

The recommended high protein low carb diet made a negative contribution to Peter's lack of progress. By consuming such a diet, Peter was forcing his body namely his kidneys, to work overtime by breaking down excess protein.

The lack of carbs was leading to the chronic fatigue, as there was not enough energy being produced to feed his muscles, which were overworked due to the excessive exercise.

Peter's guilt at neglecting his health meant that he was in the mindset of *'I must work harder to punish myself for getting into this bad way.'* He came to see the exercises as the cleansing of past sins believing that if he threw himself into recovery he would be justly rewarded with good health and the shedding of weight.

The high volume of activity placed such demand on primarily his liver that his body was demanding more calories than ever before. He would be hungry at all hours of the night and waking up at various intervals to eat unable to keep tags on how much he had consumed from one day to the next.

His diet was nutritious but the balance of meals was

heavily biased towards high levels of protein. This combined with keeping no record of food consumed, was another salient factor in limiting his success and hampering his prolonged arduous efforts.

In terms of the marathon endurance style workouts, Peter was in health terms attempting to build Rome in a day, a nigh on impossible feat.

Outcome

Sharing a short cab ride across town, Peter and I became acquainted. He told me his story almost as though he had given up on himself and accepted his state of poor health, as 'just the way it is'.

Describing how he felt he was too riddled with minor injuries ever to become healthy and slim, he had written himself off.

I explained my method for getting people healthy in the quickest, easiest way backed up by scientific research and the tools to get them to where they want to be. He was both intrigued and skeptical at my casual, confident approach to his story of disappointment.

In response to Peter's question on his efforts so far, I held no punches in giving him my views on the type of boot camp regime he had signed up to.

"All the wrong messages in terms of training volume and diet." I said. "But certainly not the end of the road for you and never too late to turn your life around."

When I said goodbye to Peter, I was not sure I would see him again.

Two weeks later, he called asking if I could design a physical training program along with a diet to regain health and lose weight.

First off, I ascertained the types of exercises Peter could do that did not impact upon his injuries. His ankles and knees were still in a bad way from the previous regime.

We settled on just two simple exercises involving the upper body, The *Air Punch Drill and Supported Uppercut and Hook*, leaving his ankle and knee joints out the equation.

I explained to Peter that upon waking he could drink a little water before immediately undertaking 10 minutes of constant cardio work. I emphasized the need for this to take place on an empty stomach and for each exercise to incorporate a fixed number of repetitions or a fixed time period. I told him he needed to do only 10 minutes, which at first he refused to believe.

"I will barely have warmed up in that time," he said.

I told him to trust me.

Next we looked at the diet. This would consist of 70% carbs 20% protein and 10% fiber in the form of vegetables. Also, he would eat as soon as he felt hungry and not skip any meals, as this hinders fat loss. We discussed how and when he should eat and portion sizes.

A week later I received a phone call from an ecstatic Peter.

"I can't believe it," he said. "I've lost 14 pounds doing hardly any cardio at all"

"By hardly any at all, I believe you mean 10 minutes a day before breakfast."

"Yeah, but that's hardly any at all."

A month later Peter had lost a further 32lbs in body fat using just the simple straightforward method I had shared with him. His blood results indicated a massive improvement in terms of bringing his cholesterol into a normal range, cutting his risk of diabetes and his blood pressure had normalized. His colleagues were complimenting him on his appearance, as he looked so much younger.

"With every compliment, I feel like weeping inside." He confided in me.

Looking good meant that he felt good about his future and all the new and exciting possibilities.

Today Peter weighs 170 pounds and no longer works as a taxi driver. He is able to run several kilometers with relative ease and remains faithful to his 10 minutes cardio before breakfast. He looks back to those days when playing with his grandson left him breathless, almost with disbelief.

Peter now works alongside me, encouraging and teaching others the principles and tools for obtaining optimum health. It is an honor working alongside Peter, as his enthusiasm and passion, combined with his great testimonial continues to inspire and transform lives.

CHAPTER THREE

The Power of the Mind

"By the right choice and true application of
thought man ascends to the divine perfection"
James Allen

WITH THE INFINITE AND OMNIPOTENT POWER of the mind we create our outer world. Whatever we furnish in the garden of our mind will take root, blossoming into physical being, the quality of our thinking, which in turn, dictates our reality.

The brain, which houses the mind, is known as the 3lb universe. It contains within it a power that lies largely untapped, capable of achieving what at first may seem impossible. It is the ultimate problem solver.

A computer might have the capacity to outsmart the brain in a multitude of mathematical or strategic instances but in initiative, creativity, intuition and the ability to weigh and measure critical factors the brain is far superior.

This chapter is about what the human mind can do when you set it on the right path.

If you want to achieve your goal of optimal health and vitality along with the best fat loss, *which I know you do*, then, your mind needs to maximize its potential. It needs to be free, unraveled from insecurity, corruption and despair and able to acknowledge its immeasurable power.

The Law of the Mind

Whatever you choose to focus your mind on, it will expand for you. If you focus your mind on a problem it will grow larger in size in proportion to the focus you place upon it. Choose to focus instead, on a solution to the problem, you will find the solution expands in relation to the focus.

On identifying a problem, the way forward is to immediately ask, what is the best and most efficient solution to this problem? Focus your mind on *solving* the problem. This makes you more valuable to yourself and the people around you.

Choosing to implement this simple change as opposed to getting stuck in a mental loop liberates the mind and increases your skill in problem solving.

The tools in this section used properly and consistently will catapult you to the top of your game. Get this part right and the rest of the fat loss process is a push over.

Positivity

"Be positive no matter what"
Les Brown

Positivity is the ability to be optimistic and constructive.
To *be* positive, is a conscious choice.

All of us contain the divine force of positivity. It is there we have it within our human DNA. All we need to do is let it in.

"Hello Positivity, you look great today and goodbye Negativity, Despair and Self-loathing"

You know how it is everybody wants to know the positive person. The one who makes you feel good about yourself, who can always find a bright side now matter how hard the rain is coming down.

Why?

Because 'Positivity' begets 'Positivity' just as 'Like' attracts 'Like'.

Learning to become positive does not happen overnight. It is something you need to work at and coming up against knocks and obstacles on the way is the best way you are going to learn.

There are always people who will try to put you down and belittle your achievements not to mention Life itself, which loves to share interruptions and occasional catastrophes. Learning to see setbacks and disappointments as par of the course as opposed to personal affronts will enable you to make positivity your default mode.

Being overweight encourages feelings of negativity towards oneself. This is an understandable state of mind but you need to know that you have the power within you to switch your state from negativity to positivity.

As Leonardo da Vinci said: *"One can have no smaller or greater mastery than mastery of oneself"*.

To acquire a permanently positive state requires daily, diligent practice.

Learn to become sentinel over your thoughts making negative thoughts redundant, edging them out by using positivity to vanquish their existence.

Positive thought can be likened to the light of the sun. With each dawn the light effortlessly vanquishes darkness. Refuse to partake in activities that bring you down, such as gossiping, backbiting or the disparagement of others either at home or at work. Know that when you do you are giving away vital energy force for greatness and cheapening your divine nature. Take a firm stance on refusing to judge others.

"Judge not less ye be judged" (Matthew 7:1-3). When you act as a judge over others you are simply attracting the same negative judgment on to yourself.

The most dynamic people in the history of the world know that above all other attributes positivity is the foundation for their success. This is regardless of what problem or obstacle is placed before them.

Create your own positivity morning ritual to psychologically pump yourself up.

On first waking perform a series of positivity affirmations (*see below*) prior to moving onto your 10 minutes of cardiovascular exercises, as outlined in the previous chapter.

The Physical benefits of Positivity

Our body consists of 75% water even our bones are 35% water.

It is known scientifically to be the most receptive of the four elements.

Experiments in Japan by scientist, Masaru Emoto, have been conducted in order to discover whether the molecular structure of water can be altered using nothing more than the power of thought or intention. Using an electro microscope to study the molecular structure of the water, experimenters exposed water to various genres of music. On playing classical music to the water, the frozen molecules formed beautiful, elegant structures, a delight to behold. Conversely when exposed to heavy metal the structure was more complicated and chaotic.

The Water Rice Experiment involved taking three identical jars and filling each with the same amount of water, then adding an identical fixed quantity of rice and placing them 30 cm apart on a level surface.

Each morning, to Jar One the message, 'Thank you' was repeatedly said out loud. To Jar Two, the message was, "You Idiot" while Jar Three was completely ignored.

After 15 days, the rice contained in Jar One, emitted a pleasant fragrance from the rice. The rice in Jar Two turned black. In Jar Three, the one that was ignored, the rice was decomposed.

From such an experiment, one could derive that positive intention or positivity is the supreme force upon matter and negativity a destructive force, whilst, indeed, the most destructive force of all, is being ignored.

What this experiment illustrates beyond conventional knowledge is that in order to be the best we can be we must utilize the divine miracle of positive intention in our life. There is no downside to choosing this as it can only reap benefits.

Top Tip for Positivity

The Law of Substitution states that the conscious mind can only maintain one focus at any time, positive or negative. Knowing this means we are in the position to instantly switch from one mind-set to another – from negative to positive. Switching so rapidly might at first feel unfamiliar, as we break old negative mental patters but practise it for a few days and you will note the dramatic change for the better.

When people try to engage you in negative chat, reengage them attempting to bring positivity back into the conversation. When you do this, you are maintaining the powerful imaging faculty of your mind on the positive as well as protecting your mental and emotional energy levels.

Always be consciously focused on things you want both in your mind and in in the conversations you choose to have.

Self Esteem

"Because one believes in oneself, one does not try to convince others. Because one is content with oneself, one does not need others' approval. Because one accepts oneself, the whole world accepts him or her."

Lao Tzu

Self esteem can be described as one's ability to view themselves as competent in dealing with the challenges of life, combined with being able to view oneself as one worthy of happiness.

Self Efficacy

The first component of this is self efficacy. This means the ability to think for one's self as well as being able to direct one's own life. To know if one has a high level of self efficacy is simply to know that one has the ability to deal with the challenges of life, someone who is undaunted by negative setbacks or circumstances.

Self Respect and Self Worth

The second component of self esteem is self respect or self worth, feeling within that you have a right above all else to be happy.

Self esteem is the best buddy of positivity, although it is possible to be positive alongside having low self esteem. Self esteem has been proven to govern success. One can have a superior education, excellent technical knowledge, access to unrivalled resources but if they have low self esteem they will come to flounder in the best and most well laid out plans. This is because they lack the belief and self worth. Inside – through it all, they think of themselves as nothing.

Conversely you have individuals who lack education and technical knowledge as well as having no resources, but they have a high level of self esteem enabling them to act in faith towards their dreams. Examples abound of those who have been unable to read or write yet became incredible leaders in business, sport, religion. Why? High self esteem.

Self esteem comes down to how much you like yourself as well as how much you feel deep down you deserve happiness and fulfillment in your life.

Self Esteem and Body Weight

For a wide range of people with a weight issue, low self esteem is a common factor. Lack of self esteem generally goes hand in hand with being overweight. What is good here (*note the positive thinking*), is that your level of self esteem can be taken from low to high by diligently practicing just a few specific affirmations every morning and evening – *see below.*

Over time you will find that feeling better about yourself will make others around you feel better too. This is in turn will fuel you to feel *even* better about yourself and so on. Remember positivity begets positivity. You will begin to create this positive chain of cause and effect within your life initiated by you!

High esteem finds its way into all aspects of your life. Your confidence increases, the quality of your relationships with other people heightens, you begin to make wiser choices, as you believe in obtaining the best for yourself and those around you. Family, friends, colleagues sensing this shift whether consciously or subconsciously will hone into your energy and simply by liking to be with you, will assist you in obtaining your goals.

Performing affirmations that ignite your self esteem on a consistent daily basis will blast you into the orbit of success. The momentum will enable you to pour yourself into the cardio and nutritional requirements with confidence, faith and gusto. As you begin to shed body fat, you will find your self esteem increases even more and life takes on a whole new meaning.

You are the enabler in your life.

Human beings are extremely susceptible to the vibrational frequencies of the people they encounter, even without saying a word we have this innate ability to sense how another is feeling almost like an internal antenna receiving sympathetic vibes. When you have cultivated your self esteem to a high level, other people will feel the positivity emanating from your presence. In return, you will have the ability to sense others' low self esteem and pump it up. This could be in the form of a compliment or a gesture of kindness. This is making a transfer of positive energy from yourself to the person in need, causing the mirror effect whereby they receive a self esteem boost which in turn further boosts your own self esteem, and thus the cycle of positivity.

As you perpetuate this positive cycle of increasing your self esteem as well as looking and feeling great you know that the only one who can stop you is *you*.

The giant of philosophy, Friedrich Nietzsche states:

"You must learn to climb mountains until you can climb no further, then you must climb upon your own head!"

Each of us has our own unique mountains to overcome in the form of goals and obstacles but ultimately, the greatest challenge is conquering ourselves.

High self esteem is what makes the difference between being poor, average or good at what one does and being an absolute runaway success. If you wish to break away from the pack, then work on your self esteem. Make it a priority to cultivate on a daily basis and protect it from anything or anyone that attempts to suck its lifeblood.

Buying diet advice, training or fat loss products to solve body weight issues is a waste of time, as it detracts from the root of the issue, which is namely your self esteem, the logic is there but the outcome will be ineffectual. What needs to be addressed is the issue that *leads* to you being overweight in the first place.

Could it be a throwback from the past? An unhappy childhood perhaps? Were you bullied, or told consistently that you were *not* good enough? Do you feel inadequate within? Are you unhappy now? Is it a current relationship? Are you lonely?

Working through the reasons *why* is vital in understanding how to raise self esteem. If you can understand *why*, you can work better in focusing your energies on increasing it.

Persistently pumping up self esteem can be likened to pumping hot air into an air balloon. The more air that enters, the higher the balloon ascends attracting the gaze of onlookers, struck by its brilliance. This balloon represents all the dimensions of your life. Many balloons deflate before even getting the chance to inflate.

A person with high self esteem encounters setbacks but they bounce back because they see everything as a learning experience, another opportunity to grow and refine their methods. If you have low self esteem, every setback is considered a severe blow.

The ability to see each failure as the chance to grow, to do better next time, is a necessary part of obtaining self esteem. Getting up again after every failed attempt and having another bloody good go.

This is an unwritten rule that people with high self esteem intrinsically know. Implementing this idea within your life means that with each setback your self esteem grows, you fail, you learn, you go again, After a while, you begin to gather a pool of positive momentum driving you forward. In essence, you become your own force of nature as a problem is converted from something previously perceived as negative to a stepping-stone closer to your goal What does not kill one only makes one stronger.

So do not be afraid to fail, instead be afraid not to try, try, and try again.

As you begin to make steady progress towards your goal each day and each week witnessing the weight loss on the scales as well as the all new fresh appearance in the mirror, this will also feed directly into your self esteem, as you become more valuable by having the ability to be whomever or whatever you wish to be.

Top Tip for Self Esteem

Write down 10 things you like about yourself; past or present, awards, achievements, kindnesses, your eyes, your laugh – anything. As you approach your target of 10 you might be getting close to running out of thoughts. Don't stop. Just this act of pushing mental iron will force you into a positive state regardless of how low you feel.

Keep this list somewhere safe and refer to it whenever

you feel the need for a psychological boost.

Bonus Tip

Give something away to someone else every single day, it could be a smile, it could be letting someone in front of you at the shopping till, it could be sending a card to an old friend or phoning a relative. It is amazing how a random act of kindness works no end for boosting self esteem.

Emotions

"When a man is at pray to his emotions he is at the mercy of fortune"

Spinoza

As stated by the philosopher, Spinoza, a person lacks the ability to govern ones self if they are occupied by their emotions on a frequent and persistent basis. The emotions contained within all of us have the overwhelming power to make us irrational, unreasonable and act out of impulse. In essence our emotions can in some cases cause us to behave in our most primitive modes and as stated above put us at the mercy of fortune.

Emotions set humans apart from the animal kingdom and are an indisputable part of who we truly are. Indeed,

"If you take away emotions what difference remains I do not say between a man and a beast." Said *Roman philosopher, Cicero.*

When a person finds himself frequently reacting emotionally to his environment, he is in a weakened state whether he outwardly externalizes the emotion or holds it in, either way, how he feels is dictated by his environment and thus he is not able to act with a moderate level of rationality and equanimity. In short his own emotions are overwhelming his capacity to operate at his optimal level.

The philosopher, Aristotle observed that man should endeavor to neither have too much emotion nor a complete lack of emotion within life but rather a proper balance of the emotions to truly live well.

Emotional detachment can occur in people who within a period of their lives have been neglected, abused or suffered mental or physical trauma. The signs or symptoms can include violent outbursts, self harm and harm to others and a sense of being possessed internally with emotions that rear up in the person unexpectedly.

This impacts negatively upon relationships as well as ones ability to navigate and communicate effectively in the world. It also serves to isolate individuals from developing and maintaining healthy, happy relationships.

The great spiritual teacher as well as medical doctor, Deepak Chopra, describes our emotions as being like that of clouds in the sky, 'they appear solid and look permanent but clouds just like our emotions drift away in given time'.

Using Emotions To Your Advantage

A How-To Guide

As described earlier our emotions are a powerful force

contained within all of us. They can be likened to an internal energy rich weather system that can work for or against us depending on how we respond to them.

Emotions have the power to immobilize us rendering us powerless, but they also have the power to energize and strengthen us if channeled correctly into action.

In order that we can tap into the energy of our emotions we need firstly to recognize what external or internal factors are causing the generation of the given emotion. This could be a past negative experience in the form of a memory or it could be an individual who upsets you.

Once you are able to identify the source of the emotion you are half the way towards channeling it into an action that is beneficial to you achieving your goal. By witnessing, observing and acknowledging its existence you can take the emotion whether it be anger, sadness, guilt and in some cases joy and make a conscious decision to pour the energy straight into your daily health practices.

This might come in the form of diligently writing out the affirmation of your goal, the performance of your 10 minutes morning cardio or accurate implementation of your diet.

This method of converting emotion into a catalyst for ongoing improvement is a superior use of the powerful forces contained within us. Instead of being a captive or slave to our emotions allowing them to limit us, we make them work for us by means of a mental alchemy, a power source.

You often hear people saying that they lack motivation and go hunting around for a product or trainer to get them going. What they need to realize they have, however, is an abundance of energy all around them as well as within them. All of us are intrinsically powerful beyond measure.

The motivation is everywhere. It could be the school teacher who told you that you were not good enough, the parent or sibling who belittled you by making you feel inferior or perhaps the ex-partner who took away your confidence by means of their lies, whatever the case, take the energy of upset, hurt and disappointment and fire it into setting a goal.

Emotions in Relation to food

"Change in diet will not help the man who will not change his thoughts, when a man makes his thoughts pure he no longer desires impure food"
James Allen

How emotions affect our dietary patterns is a vital component in understanding how we are to unlock our full potential for health vitality and fat loss.

Emotion influences the manner in which people form relationships with food and certain types of food. One study carried out on emotion in relation to people on diets discovered that when individuals felt strong emotional urges and they repressed or ignored them, the likelihood of coming off their diet and binging on poor quality, unhealthy food, rocketed. It found that people were using food to regulate their emotional states, commonly known as "comfort eating".

Four Classic Examples of Emotional Eating

1. The Midnight or Late Night Feast

So another successful day of completing all the necessary requirements for losing fat and becoming healthy and for our efforts we are reaping the fantastic rewards we deserve. How proud we are of our accomplishments.

With bedtime approaching, we are settling down ready to go to sleep, when we are hit by the overwhelming urge to raid the fridge for food that we well know will take us backwards next time we hit the scales. 'Come on, though', we say to ourselves, 'just a little won't harm us. No one will ever know and we don't want to be hungry in the night.'

This self deception is coupled with the fact we consume food in secret when nobody is around to see us. This serves to reinforce the false notion that it won't count when we hit the scales. After all we deserve a treat once in a while right?

These justifications may sound rational and reasonable but what is going on here is that the 'occasional treat' becomes a 'regular treat', a 'nightly treat' that, as it ingratiates itself, serves to stunt our progress and weaken our resolve to keep plugging away at the diet until in the end there is a sort of 'Us' and 'Them' situation going on. 'Us' being the secret eaters and 'Them' being the demands of the diet.

Emotional late night eating along with its absurd reasoning and the strong sense of entitlement links directly to the inner child living in all of us, the child who acts out of impulse, demanding immediate gratification.

2. The Comfort Indulging after the Conflict

So again, you are making daily progress by doing what is necessary to get the fantastic results you deserve, using the cardio combined with faithfully implementing the diet, gathering momentum and growing in confidence. It seems that you are unstoppable.

All of a sudden, however, someone or something knocks you out of alignment and you plummet back into the cycle of old negative habits, your goal is jeopardized.

Despite all of your best efforts, when life throws you a spanner, the external conflict causes an internal stirring of emotions.

It is at these times that we can seek comfort to regain a sense of balance. Enter the role of food but not just any food, junk food, food that brings no benefit in the terms of health but is packed full of comforting ingredients; a liter of ice cream, a few bars of chocolate, a slab of cheese. Often it is foods that brought comfort in your childhood or that you were perhaps restricted from eating and you now have the power to eat. These are the foods that you most crave.

We are all creatures of habit and reverting back to something that connects us with our past is deeply rooted within the human psyche and closely related to our animal instinct. In times of uncertainty we seek refuge in familiarity, in this case, food.

3. The Shopping Spree Pig Out

Suppressing our inner desire for 'bad' food as well as maintaining our diet also has a secondary effect, namely that we crave a type of substitution in order to fill the void. This substitute is the desire for a product or set of products that we believe will satisfy us. These might come in material form be it new clothing, electrical devices or other such items that we think will complete and satiate our inner emotional desire.

We go on a shopping spree for that special product or set of products and gratify our desire but now we are hungry again. We are now into the cross over effect whereby we want to maintain the 'high from the buy'. Buying stuff feels good. Eating stuff feels good too, we like this emotion we are feeling. So, we pig out because we want the good feeling to last. The only problem is, it lasts only the length of time we are consuming. At some stage or other, we have to come back down again. This is a negative gratification response.

4. The Automatic Indulge Meant Response

This classic form of emotional eating may sound complex, but can be best likened to the effects of coming off a diet.

We are on a diet we know that clearly works from the visible results both on the scales and our fantastic look and feel. For some mysterious reason, however, we find ourselves indulging in a high sugar splurge at the same time, like clockwork, every evening. We feel powerless to resist temptation. Our pattern of behavior could be described as automatic or even robotic in nature.

What happens is an automatic response to stimuli or stimulation, causing us to break our chain of healthy meals with the piece of cake, the doughnut, the chocolate bar, or the ice cream.

The stimuli that precedes the splurge could be the theme tune to a for example, soap opera or regular sporting event that excites within you the desire to have that large slice of gateau. Regardless of the specific type of stimuli your response remains automatic.

Ivan Pavlov was a Russian scientist who lived between 1849 and 1936 and was a recipient of the Nobel Prize in physiology for his study on the digestive systems of dogs. He stumbled upon a form of behavioral conditioning that found dogs producing saliva long before they were presented with any food. This was in preparation for the food because they had seen the lab coat wearer, and it was routinely the lab coat wearer who fed the dogs.

They had learned to associate the appearance of the lab coat with the imminent arrival of food. Pavlov named this discovery *Classic Conditioning*.

The same happened when Pavlov rang a bell prior to feeding time.

The conclusion of these various experiments was that regardless of the type of stimuli, so long as it is consistent, the physiological response is always the same.

We are all victims of what has been coined the *Pavlovian Response* responding to the sound or appearance of specific stimuli to reach for the sweet.

By having an awareness of this feature of comfort eating is the starting point for controlling it.

Top Tip For Emotion and Food

Use a phone or tablet device to keep a basic journal entitled "Room for Improvement." Write a few sentences to describe the obstacle or issue you are experiencing in terms of your attitude to food. Be specific including the time and date and how you feel about the particular issue. Review your sentences after seven days and look for a pattern or set of circumstances that lie at the root of the problem. Once you have established a cause, the problem can be solved quickly and easily by either avoiding the particular set of circumstances or by employing a strategy to implement in case it arises. Have you someone you can speak to about your concerns? Be prepared to wear your heart on your sleeve when discussing how you feel with other people. You will be amazed at how much people will want to assist you in achieving your goals.

Bonus Tip

Write a list of your burdens and worries and then as an impulse exercise, write a snapshot solution. Snapshot solution means the first answer that pops into your head generally within 10 seconds. Research has shown that this "snapshot solution" is almost always 100% accurate in terms of eliminating the burden/worry.

Your list should contain up to 10 burdens/worries along with their accompanying solutions. Separate each one on to its own piece of paper.

Each of the following three rituals will cleanse you of your burden/worry.

1. Burning the paper
2. Casting it into a river or stream
3. Burying it in the garden.

Try and put emotional content into the ritual by reading out loud the burden/worry adding emotion to the words as you speak out loud. This will bring added power to the cleansing ritual. Now, simply do away with each piece of paper until all are gone. You will feel fantastic when rid of all your burdens.

Conquering Fear

"If there is no enemy within then the enemies outside can do you no harm"
African Proverb

Fear is a deeply unpleasant, disturbing feeling brought about by the presence or eminent threat of danger. We may share some of the more common fears with others but in the deep recesses of our minds we have fears that only we know. These fears inhabit our minds like old junk that we refuse to dispose of. As a result of this, we allow them a free pass, permitting them to circulate within our imagination affecting everything we do. They hold us back, from trying new things to impounding our relationships. Fear whether conscious or subconscious could be likened to an old school master watching over our actions and waiting to punish us for stepping out of line or away from our comfort zone.

As the old African proverb above states if there is no enemy within, the enemies outside can do us no harm. Fear is not an external but an internal conflict. Its roots lie in childhood conditioning namely, the fear that we can't do something and the fear that we won't do it well enough.

Contained within each of our fears is great treasure. By great treasure we mean, when a fear is overcome and conquered the powerful force contained within it, the *treasure*, is released. This creates a mental expansion that makes us stronger. Conquering our fears is the foundation of growth as well as the expansion of our power base.

Regardless of the type of person you are or the fears you have, the internal mechanism is the same, namely the feeling of being afraid that you must learn to overcome. There will be some pain in doing so and discomfort to contend with but this is perfectly normal and all part of the process.

Write down anything and everything you are afraid of no matter how trivial and remember your list of fears is unique and belongs only to you.

Once you have your list it is time for positive action.

Choose one fear and break it down into five to ten small steps. At the beginning you may only manage to perform a couple of the steps before stopping, but simply endeavor to add an extra step the next time. This gradual ebbing away of your individual fears bit by bit is the road to becoming master of your destiny.

As you cross each individual fear off your list, you gain more fear-conquering experience until an internal transition takes place and you learn to become accustomed to the sensation of fear, enabling you to use it as a force for action.

In ancient Japan, before a battle, the Samurai would prepare by meditating on the sensation of being torn to pieces by arrows and swords. They would imagine meeting a gory end. This simple mental technique cleansed their minds of any doubts and fears as they had already accepted the reality that they could be slaughtered and therefore had no fear for it. This meant that when they entered the battlefield, they were able to annihilate their adversaries with efficient finesse.

The Samurai as well as being great warriors were also great philosophers and had thought long on using the full power of their minds before the battle. The simple technique of imagining the worst before conquering a fear is highly effective. Choose a fear to overcome and before embarking on surmounting it, take a few minutes beforehand to contemplate the worst case scenario. Now set about taking the five to ten action steps to conquering your fear.

Fear can sharpen our skills allowing us to push beyond our limits taking us to new heights. The American President, Franklin D Roosevelt stated, *"There is nothing to fear except fear itself,"* therefore in order to taste the rich rewards of life, we must become acquainted with our fears and like only human beings can, embrace them.

As you plough forward conquering your own unique

list of fears and checking them off as you go, you will find that after a short period you will revisit your previous fears and find some of them barely fears at all. This is because, by conquering the fear you have grown strong, an internal shift has occurred within you and you are no longer afraid of what tormented you. Coming to understand that fear can be transcended by a series of action steps, will empower you for the rest of your life.

Top Tip for Fear

Rationalise It. Firstly gain perspective on the fear you have. Most fear emanates from being locked into only one future possibility. Remembering the 'truth of infinite possibilities' will enable you to gain perspective on your fears and rework your mind into either thinking around them or seeking other equally likely outcomes. Thinking yourself out of a fear is both liberating and powerful as you realize you never need to be trapped.

Look your fear in the eye. You are not scared of it. Write it down, screw it up and throw it in the bin. Accept it as just that, a fear. By doing this, you will overcome the negative aspect of fear and empower yourself to overcome it.

Believe you can do it. By overcoming one fear, once, you will have provided yourself with the tools to overcome fear twice, three times and so on. Self-belief comes from challenging yourself to do the impossible and achieving your aim. From this, you build on overcoming other fears.

Remember, once upon a time, you never had this fear. Fear is a learned emotion. There was a time when you never feared what you most fear now. If you can learn the emotion, you can unlearn it. Fear is simply a feeling and the only power it has, is what we feed it. If it is unfed, it will not survive. Facing up to your fear, spending time with it, accepting it, is the path to overcoming it.

The Power of Affirmations

"The Body is the servant of the mind it obeys the operations of the mind"
James Allen

An affirmation is as a direct command delivered to the conscious and subconscious mind in order to illicit a specific response from the mind. The nature and type of response relates directly to the type of command given as well as the emotional content of the command.

This next part will cover the affirmations for you to perform, the reason for performing each one, along with the manner and frequency with which they are to be performed for maximum positive results.

Remember, the beauty of performing these affirmations is that they begin to work immediately.

All of the affirmations listed are best performed **first thing on waking**, as this window of mental opportunity has been scientifically proven to be when the mind is most responsive.

Also, the affirmations are to be repeated in the same way **just before you drift off to sleep**. What this does is insert the affirmation/command into the mind on a conscious level, and reinforces it when you drift into deep sleep. The net effect of these new positive affirmations/commands circulating around your subconscious mind is profound. As you rise and sleep performing your standardized affirmations morning and night, your life will begin to take on a dynamic that will filter on through to you expecting the best from your relationships, your finances, your lifestyle and so on.

Within a few short few weeks you will find that with the daily diligent practice of positive affirmations, optimal fat loss is only the beginning of your fantastic new life.

By performing a specific set of key affirmations, you are essentially enabling yourself to remain objective when life throws obstacles and challenges your way, which inevitably it will. Positive affirmations will enable you to keep your mind cool and calm and in control by finding the good in every situation.

The Affirmations

When you begin to utter your first affirmations they will sound foreign. You may feel a sense of internal discomfort. This is perfectly normal and to be expected even welcomed. The reason I use the word 'welcomed' is because if the affirmations did NOT feel alien then you would have no need to perform them, as you must already possess the necessary mental components. Take comfort therefore in their strangeness, knowing you are in the right place for change.

Perform each individual affirmation **ten times** out

loud. Each affirmation **must** contain emotional content spoken with conviction and purpose.

Your immediate objective should be to form the longest unbroken chain of affirmation days possible. Keep note of the number of days you manage to accumulate without a break and if you do stop for any reason, simply start again only this time endeavoring to beat your previously unbroken chain.

Below are the affirmations that will make you positive, heighten your self esteem and make you master of your emotions:

The first and most important:

I LIKE MYSELF

I like myself.

Say it a few times, get used to how it sounds, feel it when you say it, believe it because this is going to be your main affirmation.

The affirmation, 'I like myself', yields the greatest rewards in terms of supercharging your mind. The ability to 'like yourself' is directly related to your ability to succeed in all aspects of your life.

Brian Tracy, lead figure in self development, refers to the 'I like myself' affirmation as the single overall statement above all else that will dictate a person's success. He ranks it higher than a person's intelligence and status in the world. It is, he believes, the magic ingredient for a positive life.

Other Affirmations:

Positivity
I have incredible strength within

I am confident and kind

I am valuable

Self Esteem
I do my best and expect the best

I am valuable

The Emotions
I am sentinel over my emotions

I pour emotion into positive action

I love my work

Conquering fear
I can do it

I am strong

I am unstoppable

The Law of Attraction
What you expect from your life, you will achieve in your life, this is the law of attraction. If you believe your life will be hard or unhappy or difficult, it will be. Expect success, happiness and achievement and by the law of attraction, you will make it happen. The universe is made up of energy that constantly emits frequency. Everything is made up of energy waves. Energy waves are attracted to other energy waves of the same frequency. If you,

therefore, put out positive energy waves, you will attract positive energy waves. It is the magnetic power of the universe drawing similar energies together. By repeating positive statements, you are bringing into your life what you repeat in your mind. Make the power of the universe work for you.

Top Tip for Affirmations

When going through your morning affirmations program use a smart phone or tablet device and switch audio description on, then increase the speech rate to around 60 or 70 percent. Go over each affirmation 10 times as described earlier only instead of reading through 10 of each affirmations you can quickly skim over them with your finger whilst the device speaks them out loud. Use headphones if necessary so as not to disturb anyone. What might have taken 10 minutes or more now takes around two. In this small amount of time, you are mentally pumped up and primed and ready to smash through your goals, starting with cardio.

Recap:

Positive thinking begets positive thinking.

People are drawn to those who have a bright outlook.

Self Esteem is intrinsic to some people. Others need to find it.

With self esteem, you can bounce back from all life knocks.

Identifying your emotions enables you to act upon them.

You can switch negative emotions into positive emotions.

There is no greater fear than fear itself. To overcome fear, you need to mentally train your brain to consider the worst that can happen.

You need to write down your fears, which causes you to face up to them.

Facing up to fears works to diminish them.

Case Study

"As within, so without"

Saint Francis of Assisi

Sara's Story

Sara was 34 years old, 300 pounds and worked in a bank. She had been overweight most of her life and as a result, lacked confidence and self esteem. Growing up an only child, Sara was never wanted, 'a mistake' her single mother, an estate agent, told her on an almost daily basis. Sara's mother craved attention for herself but rarely shared it with Sara.

When a new husband came onto the scene, Sara was completely sidelined and had to fend for herself from her early teens. It was around this time that she got into bad eating habits.

Her mother used to restrict her from eating particular types of food because she would 'get fat' and so Sara would sneak junk food up to her room and eat by herself, hiding all the evidence.

She was living alone but still binge eating at night, which led her to hate herself and feel fat and unattractive. Her loneliest time was in the evenings when watching the soaps. These always prompted her to get up and go to her fridge. She ate solidly for the duration of the program then went to bed.

Sara had never experienced a happy relationship with a man or particularly had any friends. Due to her lifestyle and lack of self worth, she was often moody at work and so generally avoided by her colleagues for 'bringing people down'. To deal with the loneliness, she would eat more and despite attempts in the past, was unable to break the negative cycle.

Interpretation

Due to an unhappy childhood, Sara developed a negative attitude to food, in that it needed to be eaten in secret. As a child, food was restricted so she never had the opportunity to learn how to control her own appetite, her relationship with food simply being the chance to 'rebel' against her mother. Food for Sara had become only comfort, a way of making herself feel better, of empowering her and as a substitute for loneliness. As she was never particularly loved as a child she did not value herself, worse, she hated herself. This was why people avoided her, because her outlook on life was so negative and people do not like to be made depressed.

Outcome

I had the fortune of meeting Sara. Her initial reaction was to close in on herself and make no attempt to converse but sensing sadness about her (and a professional interest), I persisted. She told me she had never considered the link between her childhood and her weight assuming she just 'enjoyed her food.' It became apparent early on in the conversation that I was dealing with a very depressed person, someone who was continually putting herself down and didn't have much on the horizon to look forward to.

After a reasonable amount of time, I told her of my

Affirmation program, explained how powerful the mind is in shifting self perceptions and how quick the process is to start feeling positive about oneself. I could tell she had never really known what 'positivity' was.

I dispatched her with my program of cardio exercises and a list of affirmations to be done first thing in the morning and last thing at night. I explained to her the importance of due diligence and consistency and we discussed a suitable diet.

A few days later, I received a call from Sara, telling me that she had started really well but a bad day at work caused her to have a 'fridge binge'. I told her this can be expected, old habits die hard, but I emphasized the importance of an unbroken chain of affirmations. We agreed to speak again 14 days later when hopefully, she would have had no blips in her treatment.

In fact, we spoke 18 days later and her affirmation chain was still intact. She had been completing the cardio exercises religiously and sticking (more or less) to the diet. I could tell by her voice that she was uplifted. She had a bouncy lilt in the way she spoke and she laughed – I had never heard her laugh before. She informed me that she had been invited out to Friday night drinks with her colleagues not that she would drink because she was trying to achieve her goal of losing 110 pounds.

A week later, she called to tell me that she was going on a date with one of her male colleagues. "He likes me because he thinks I am good fun." She said sounding a little skeptical. She said she had stopped listening to Radio 4 at night to eliminate the 'fridge binge' trigger and simply by sleeping better and waking up lighter and more refreshed, she found the day ahead an exciting prospect.

Two years on and Sara is a completely changed person. She has even made up with her mother and is able to speak about her now without looking sad. She has a partner who loves jogging and sailing and she was just planning an island-hopping holiday in Greece. She looks great, she is slim, smiley and still does her affirmations every day. In fact, when I asked her how she felt about herself, her answer was, "You know what, I am valuable."

CHAPTER FOUR

You Are What You Eat

Let food be about Medicine and Medicine be about food

Hippocrates

IN THE HELLENIC PERIOD WHEN it was believed the gods were responsible for mans' actions on earth, it was Hippocrates who suggested that diseases were caused by nature as opposed to the gods. Further to this, Hippocrates used diet to treat many illnesses. There has always been the belief that eating the right foods is all a body needs in order to stay fit and healthy.

A Slice of Success

We've discussed the importance of exercise and the power of the mind, now for the big one: Nutrition.

You *are* what you eat.

Let's divide this section into three mouthwatering slices:

Slice One: An understanding of eating well

Slice Two: A willingness to eat well

Slice Three: The maintaining of a healthy diet

Go on dig in, take a slice of each, there is plenty to go around. When you adopt these three components, you *will* succeed in reaching your goal.

It might seem like an enormous task. Just like eating an elephant in one sitting is an enormous task but eat a bit of an elephant every day and it is not insurmountable *(eating elephants not part of your recommended daily allowance).*

To have a bit of fun with the above three slices, let's imagine you were building your dream home.

You want it big, solid, three stories high with a large garden, swimming pool and private cinema. Sounds great. You can either build it to last with bricks and mortar and top quality timber or you can build it to crumble and rot with cotton wool, cardboard and pot plants.

It's a no brainer.

So, let's imagine you are building your dream body. You want it strong and slim, full of energy, clear skin, glossy hair and white teeth. Sounds great. You can either build it to last with a fine balance of protein, fats, fruit, fiber, carbohydrates, vitamins and minerals or you can build it to crumble and rot with stress, salt, E numbers, synthetics and who knows what else?

It's a no brainer.

Your ability to live long, well and happy is totally dependent upon the raw materials you choose to fuel that wonderful body of yours.

Eat well – live well. It is that simple. Eat unhealthily – crumble and rot.

Take heart, though, you are not alone on your journey. Never, never, never. Out there in the great big world of mass media, advertising and subliminal message sharing, there are corporations, caring and kind CEO's and pharmaceutical presidents willing you to succeed in your quest for fine health.

At every turn, we are presented with 'life changing', 'life enhancing', 'essential' products GUARANTEED to improve health and vitality and fat reduction and energy and wellbeing and 'the new you'.

Pills and liquids and gels and oils and ointments and pots and pans and waxes and cans and vials and flasks and vessels and all other words in the Thesaurus stemming from the word 'bottle' to ensure you live well.

The bad news is, these wonders on the whole DO NOT WORK. Worse, they confuse and bamboozle the consumer. We believe we are buying the 'next best thing' in health and fat loss. When it does not work, we quit using it disillusioned and find ourselves back at square one.

When the next new fangled product comes along, we try it again and surprise, surprise, it fails and then its back to the old habits.

The only loss you can expect with a vast number of fat loss, 'look good' products on the market is the loss of your hard earned cash.

In this chapter, we will uncover all the ways you can use diet to help *yourself*.

It is a chapter made up of wholesome foods you can eat, unwholesome foods you can eliminate and best of all, it is 100% GUARANTEED to be free of pills, flasks and vials.

Diets That Do No Good

First off, let's get rid of many of the anathemas relating to diet and fat loss. All of you with an interest in losing weight will be familiar with the main diets everyone is talking about:

Atkins Diet

Low Carb Diet

The Starvation Diet

The 100% Fruit Diet

Shake Diet

The Meal Delivery Diet

So, do they work?

Atkins Diet

Dr Robert Atkins, American physician and cardiologist caused tidal waves of curiosity when he rolled out his weight loss diet to the world. What he said, in a para-phrased form was, 'Folks, forget starving yourself on wilted lettuce leaves, with my diet the *Atkins Diet*, you can eat protein, lots and lots of it to your heart's content AND lose weight.'

What? You mean bacon, Yes, sausages YES, burgers, YES.

What I mean is, you can eat the whole lot AND look great.

Who wouldn't jump on that bandwagon?

This was like a dream come true for every dieter in the land. What is more, the diet works. The proof was in the protein-rich pudding and all skeptics could do was shake their heads from the sidelines.

So how does it work?

In the stomach, one of the main components for breaking down food is hydrochloric acid. Depending on the foods you eat, will depend on how much hydrochloric acid is needed and therefore, how much energy is required to break the food down. Proteins particularly animal proteins require high quantities of hydrochloric acid. It is because of the energy used in digesting proteins that the fat loss occurs. Your stomach, in a sense goes into overdrive.

Sounds good right? Using lots of energy.

Not exactly

The first downside is fatigue caused by the internal energy required to break down the protein. This can lead to side effects such as headaches, body odor, muscle cramps and even heart palpitations.

Worst off, though, are the kidneys.

Too much protein causes the kidneys to hyper filtrate as they overwork to filter the immense burden placed upon them. The body goes into stress mode, which can in turn lead to permanent kidney damage.

Combining this diet with exercise, places a tremendous burden on the body.

Nowadays, there are some variations on the *Atkins Diet* whereby certain carbs are permitted, but the basic premise is the same, excess amounts of burdensome protein.

The Low Carb Diet

This is the most popular diet for reducing fat loss. There are a number of variations to this diet, some advocate increasing protein portions in conjunction with low carbs with each meal, others advocate increasing vegetable portions in conjunction with low carbs with each meal.

Whichever variation you choose, the basic premise is the same. By substantially reducing your carb intake, your body is forced to burn fat stores.

Great news yes? Well, to a certain degree.

The human body is an incredible piece of machinery, designed to run on carbohydrates. This means that we tend to break down carbohydrates much quicker and simpler than the long process needed to break down protein. We store carbohydrates in our liver and muscles in the form of glycogen.

Glycogen from the liver is used to maintain the automatic functions of the body such as the heart, lungs and diaphragm and most importantly the brain. This means that carbs are, in a sense, the life flow and primary energy source for every organ.

Significantly reducing carbs causes the body to limit the amount of glycogen sent to the muscles in order to ensure our main organs are well served by the liver. It is a little like starving Peter to feed Paul.

The greatest human muscle bear in mind is the brain.

Limiting the amount of glycogen to the brain has an

adverse impact on our mood causing it to fluctuate in peaks and troughs in between meals as blood sugar varies from moderate to low during the course of the day as well as in the evening. This leads to sleep disturbances depending on how low the carbs have been cut.

An individual on a *Low Carb Diet*, may experience initial body fat reduction, but the drawback is that they will suffer in terms of low mood, lack of energy, zest and the ability to focus and concentrate on a particular task.

Another drawback is that the initial fat reduction is seldom maintained by the individual and this is because they have for the most part had to purge themselves to such an extent that the whole arduous process of limiting carbs has placed a huge psychological burden on their inner mental resources.

This means they invariably start implementing un-healthy foodstuffs and creeping back into old eating patterns.

The conclusion of this particular diet is that it is un-healthy not in physical terms but in psychological terms, as it serves to act as a type of stern punishment built around deprivation.

The Starvation Diet

This is an oxymoron if ever I knew one and should not really be defined as a diet at all as it does not fit the dictionary definition of a diet, but for the purposes of this book we shall classify it as such.

When someone is overweight and has been for a pro-longed period be it months, years even decades they may reach a point where they are willing to try anything to reduce body fat. Starvation, however, can be an extremely negative approach for the individual both psychologically and physically.

Firstly, there is the need to understand why someone might opt for this method. Have they, perhaps been bullied into it by someone at school, in the workplace or at home? If this is the case, we are not starting from a great place.

What you have here is a negative feeling thrust upon an individual by someone else, a huge psychological burden in terms of low mood caused by consuming zero calories for someone who is already feeling low and depleted. It is not a diet this person needs but a hug.

This is an unscientific and extreme diet method whereby the purging and denying of food becomes a form of control used by the dieter as a sort of 'cry for help' emphasizing their unhappiness and low sense of self. In essence, it becomes the one constant in their life they can control.

This type of method can be rightly categorized as a medical disorder. In some rare cases the practice of starving oneself can lead to eating disorders that warrant the use of health professionals to diagnose and treat the issue. These are usually psychologists who work alongside medical doctors.

Secondly we move on to individuals who choose this method based upon a lack of knowledge who assume that by starving themselves they can achieve low levels of body fat.

The physiological characteristics of a starvation diet much like with the carb deficient diet, causes the body to go into a standby mode thus slowing the glycogen release to non-essential parts of the body primarily the muscles. This also occurs with the starvation diet except that after the initial period of slowing down, the body goes into a survival mode. By this we mean that sensing the lack of carb input it begins to release stress hormones due to a sudden large deficit in energy from the lack of calories.

Indeed, some fat is burnt for energy, but alongside this and to compensate for the lack of nutrients coming in from food, the body begins to break down lean muscle mass in order to provide additional nutrients as well as an energy source.

Another consequence is that depending on the length of the starvation period the body can begin to use nutrients from the vital organs in order to further compensate for the lack of food. This is known as the organ reserve and relates directly to the level of nutrients contained within the organs. When we are born, our organ reserve is at its peak and slowly depletes as we age. It is important that this reserve is protected as it maintains health and vitality. Without it our whole body starts to break down.

The 100% Fruit Diet

In compiling the most common unhealthy diets, the 100% Fruit Diet seems like an unlikely candidate. Except, it is up there. Not necessarily on a par with Atkins or Low

Carb but worth a mention.

Why?

Consuming a 'fruit only' diet is not a recommended fat loss method. To understand why, first we need to go back to the way in which fruit is cultivated and produced in comparison with previous decades. Our modern agricultural processes nowadays require much larger yields in order to meet increased demands and to maximize profits. In order to achieve this, producers have devised much more powerful fertilizers and other agricultural methods. These new methods greatly increase the levels of fructose or sugar contained within the fruit. This deliberate ramping up of sugar levels means the fruit we consume today is a far cry from the same moderate to low levels of sugar found contained within fruit grown and less intensively farmed decades ago.

That is not to say it is not still healthy but that it is at risk of being more harmful to the liver and kidneys.

Consuming only fruit also increases the risk of the body developing Type-Two Diabetes, due to the increased burden of sugar. It also leads to blood sugar highs and blood sugar lows causing reduced concentration and mood swings.

The Shake Diet

By shake we mean, milkshake diet, you know the one, drink a shake for breakfast, a shake for lunch and a shake for tea for almost immediate weight loss. A decade or so ago, these were all the rage.

Everyone with any weight to spare was shaking morning, noon and dusk. With closer scrutiny of the shakes, however, they were found firstly to not be milkshakes at all but protein based derivatives of milk refined and processed into power. During this processing, flavorings and preservatives are added. These flavorings and preservatives include aspartame, a neurotoxin that excites brain cells giving the consumer a 'buzz' or temporary high that is later transferred into formaldehyde proven to lead to cancer and respiratory problems.

In addition to this there is a list of E-number preservatives that serve only to prolong shelf life and enhance artificial flavor.

More recent 'shake' products on the market are derived from soya substances, which can have an adverse affect on among other functions, the thyroid.

While slick marketing creates the aura of health, the true health benefits of slimming shakes are simply a quick fix gimmick, sinisterly addictive as in the case of aspartame and certain E numbers. Any vitamins and minerals added to these products (as advertised on the packaging) work simply to counterbalance the otherwise nutritionally bankrupt ingredients.

The Meal Delivery Diet

In recent years a new trend has swept into the diet and fitness industry known as *The Meal Delivery Diet*. For a weekly or monthly direct debit, nutritious low calorie meals are delivered to your door each day giving you the convenience of not having to prepare your own weight loss, low fat meal. A multitude of providers have entered this once niche marketplace from gourmet to basic to many in between, using words such as 'flexibility' and 'freedom.' Most claim to provide the recipient with the exact nutritional requirements to lose weight.

On examination of the range of providers, the main-stay of dishes delivered were found to be processed foods in a low calorie format, although at the high end there were some that did provide highly nutritious meals. A number of providers charged customers an astronomical mark up in terms of cost, making it wholly unrealistic for the vast majority of people attempting to lose weight.

What is on offer is essentially a processed meal delivery service organized into a calorie controlled portions, in other words, a convenience meal catering perhaps for those slightly bewildered by obtaining the quality nutrition for themselves.

The concept is largely centered upon feeding those used to processed foods thereby still offering the processed foods but for premium prices in more limited aka calorie controlled portion.

How To Lose Weight Without Having to Go To Extreme Measures

The Three-Phase Diet

All of the above diets are what we might call extreme diets expecting you to radically alter your natural association with food. Do they work? In part they might but only for as long as you can bear to implement them. After a while deprivation leads to craving and craving leads to binging and binging takes you off track perhaps never to return again.

What I am introducing is a diet that barely requires anything from you just a few tweaks here and there, to your regular meals.

As you see, this is called the **Three Phase Diet.** That sounds like a lot of phases. The good news is that 99% of people on this diet never need to advance beyond *Phase One*. This is because *Phase One* is engineered and scientifically proven to work in synergy with the cardio exercises highlighted in *Chapter Two*.

The latter phases *Two and Three* are geared towards those desiring to take their weight loss into the realms of the athlete. It is for people wishing to display their abdominal muscles; pro athletes, competitive body builders or those competing for fitness. This might be you, in which case, all you need to know is here.

The underlying principle of *Phase One, Two and Three* is *Kaizen.* This is a Japanese word that means Continuous Improvement. During the 2nd World War, Japan's national infrastructure was destroyed. In rebuilding the country, the aim was to find a way of doing so that would prove to be the most highly effective it possibly could be. They came up with the *Law of Kaizen.*

This law works by increasing the level of efficiency of a task each day by one percent. It is found this principle when applied, causes a snowball effect as it teaches those implementing it to assess what they are doing in a different way. As one percent is a small amount, it is not overly challenging to employ. It was this principle that enabled the rebuilding of Japan from its war torn knees to one of the world's most prosperous nations.

So, what has this got to do with the *Three-Phase Diet?*

Applying this law to your diet requires you simply to source, plan and prepare the specific food for your diets and then, at the end of each day ask yourself: What changes can I make or adapt to this diet in order to increase its efficiency by one percent?

The change or adaptation needs to incorporate just two things.

1. Write down the answer to this question
2. At the end of each day and when you wake up, implement the change.

Changes might include preparing your meals in one batch or buying certain foods in bulk to save time. Cooking first thing in the morning when you have time or cooking the next day's food the night before.

PHASE ONE

The Incremental Improvement Phase

How and Why and What?

THE KEY TO *Phase One* is making these five small changes.

1. The Gradual Elimination of Wheat

Removing wheat from your diet is pivotal to your weight loss program. Reducing wheat will have a huge positive impact on your life. It is the foundation for fast fat reduction. Avoiding eating wheat products also comes with major health benefits.

Wheat can raise your sugar levels as much as eating sugary desserts and sweets. U.S. based cardiologist, William R Davis is the forerunner in the anti-wheat argument. He refers to wheat as, 'a perfect, chronic poison.' *Frankenwheat* as he calls it is as addictive as many addictive drugs causing people to crave it especially in the form of junk foods.

A major factor in obesity and weight gain comes from eating wheat due to wheat containing the protein, gliadin, which is an appetite stimulator. Wheat begets wheat and wheat can increase your daily calorie count by at least 400.

2. The gradual Elimination of Dairy

Believe it or not, dairy is full of sugar. Roughly 5% of

dairy is carbohydrate. People believe they need dairy for calcium but compare the levels of calcium in milk 28% with a tin of salmon 85% calcium.

3. The introduction of Drinking only Still Water

Roughly 400 calories a day are consumed through what we choose to drink; coffee, tea, juice, wine. All of these drinks also have a major effect on your energy levels causing peaks and troughs. Drinking only water is calorie free and maintains energy levels at an equilibrium.

4. Preparation of All Meals in Advance

By preparing your meals in advance means you know how to balance the rest of your eating that day. This means that when you come in from work, tired and hungry, a healthy meal is ready to go. It is healthy and it is a great way to hold back the urge to binge on readily available, unhealthy snacks.

5. Eliminating all Processed Foods

Sorry folks but processed foods are not food. They are scientific experiments. They are genetically modified and packed with pesticides and dreamt up by people in white coats. Your body requires very little energy to break down processed food. This means that you burn less calories eating processed food that you do wholesome dishes. They are also packed full of sugar. Why? Because sugar tastes good and the more sugar we have, the more sugar we crave.

Introduce Juicing in to Your Daily diet. Have we not mentioned juicing yet?

Make Juicing Your New Best Friend

So, what do we want?

Nutrients

When do we want them?

Now!

Of course you do. Remember, your body is your best friend. Your body wants you to be in the very best shape it can be and your body is doing what it can 24 hours a day to ensure you are in maximum health. BUT, it is only as good as the raw materials you put into it. The kindest thing you can do to your body is Juice.

You want to juice once a day

Why? Your body is crying out for essential nutrients that can be readily and easily absorbed. In order to get these central building blocks of health, vitality and fat reduction you would have to consume around two to five pounds of fruit and vegetables a day and that ain't easy. Eating this amount of food would require excessive chewing as well as hours of digesting a mass of fiber simply to obtain the nutrients.

Instead of burdening your body with this quantity of fiber, a simple, quick solution is to take the fruit and vegetables and juice them all at once ideally straight after cardio first thing in the morning. The performing of cardio will have primed the body to receive and absorb the maximum amount of nutrients. Also, because by the juicing method, all the fiber is removed, your body is getting pure nutrition without putting any stress onto the digestive system.

When you juice you will feel and look fantastic as you are providing your liver with the absolute best quality material to work with. Your skin will glow with vitality, your eyes sparkle and you will be bursting with high energy and optimism. The benefits of juicing are immediate.

Below is a recipe for a juice that tastes great, is packed with nutrition in the form of vitamins, minerals and living enzymes.

Ingredients

5 Medium size carrots

4 Celery Sticks

1 Green Apple

1 Lemon

1 Thumb sized piece of ginger

Method

Top and tail the carrots and celery then cut the green apple in half and use a teaspoon to remove the seeds. Do the same with the lemon. Take your thumb-sized piece of ginger and using the teaspoon quickly, skim off the outer fibrous layer until clear.

Place all the ingredients in a bowl, quickly rinse with water and feed into your juicer.

Drink the juice immediately and do not refrigerate, as this reduces the nutritional value of the juice, It is best to develop the habit of drinking the juice at room temperature.

The carrots contain carotene which detoxifies the body and makes your skin look and feel great, the celery has a calming effect on your body and promotes muscle flexibility, the apple contains pectin, which combined with the carrot is anti cancerous, the lemon although acidic, alkalizes your liver which in turn boosts your energy levels, and finally the ginger greatly improves blood circulation whilst alleviating migraine and other types of congestion.

If you do not have a juicer and are considering purchasing one choose the one, which removes the fiber/pulp as opposed to a simple blender.

Avoid purchasing an expensive juicer as the benefits of a more expensive one are negligible, between $60 – $100 is a fair price to pay, as you will be using it everyday.

There are countless testimonials of people having suffered severe and chronic health conditions for years who as a last resort, turned to juicing daily and have discovered after just several weeks, their symptoms to disappear completely. After retaking medical tests for their previous medical condition many have found that this is cured.

Science has shown conclusively that an individual's level of nutrition directly affects their mental and emotional state. Poor nutrition in the form of processed and refined foods nearly always equal low mood, low concentration and low energy. In comparison, quality nutrition namely consuming fresh juice after cardio equals high mood, high concentration and high energy levels.

Night owls who have previously described themselves as 'rubbish in the morning' have been transformed into optimistic larks simply by doing 10 minutes of cardio followed by a freshly juiced juice.

The reality of juicing is that consuming a fresh juice each day means that you will be putting high quality nutrients into your body, which will far exceed anything you could purchase at a health food store all at a fraction of the cost.

Make juicing a daily ritual and feel the immediate benefits, also make it a social or family affair sharing your joy of blended fruit and veg. By getting others involved whilst extolling the immense benefits of consuming fresh produce, you will be celebrating good nutrition as well as further locking in the powerful habit of your new practice.

Foods To Eliminate From Your Diet

Wheat is a cereal grain originally cultivated in the Eastern Mediterranean but now grown everywhere. In 2016, there was 749 million tons of wheat produced worldwide. After maize, it is the second most cultivated crop.

Wheat, when broken down rapidly arrives in the bloodstream as glucose. Influx of glucose causes the blood sugar levels to spike. After the spike comes the equally rapid drop, which makes us hungry all over again and we find ourselves on what is known as the carbohydrate rollercoaster springing between hungry and full. This is not a reliable way to manage our weight.

Foods containing wheat

Bread

Most cereals

Pasta

Processed Dairy

This creates acidity in the gut due to current dairy farming methods. Acidity leads to inflammation, food allergies, arthritis, mood swings, depression, constipation and stress. What our bodies thrive on is an alkaline environment. When we eat foods that create acidity, the body has to work its darndest to restore optimum alkaline levels. This requires the overuse of buffer minerals such as magnesium, potassium and calcium to come across and neutralize the acid. Overuse of these minerals in this department takes them away from where they should be working, which is in keeping the body and bones strong. This puts us at higher risk of bone diseases such as osteoporosis and overworks the body.

Foods Containing Dairy

Milk

Cheese

Chocolate

Ice Cream

Yoghurt

Butter

Soy Based Products

Soy is a protein derived from an East Asian bean believed to be a significant and cheap source of protein. It was in its earliest form, planted and harvested by a major car manufacturer as a raw material used to produce paint and forms of rubber. Tasty huh?

For the body, it is highly resilient and difficult to process. This is because it is high in phytic acid, which is also known as the 'anti nutrient' because it blocks the uptake of essential minerals such as calcium, magnesium and zinc in the intestine. It is also said to block the body's naturally occurring hormonal balance by affecting the thyroid gland and can lead to a reduction in fertility for women.

Foods Containing Soy

Sweets

Most chocolate contains soy lecithin used as a cheap
    filling agent.

Some energy bars

Mayonnaise

Peanut butter

Margarine

Vegetarian meat substitutes

Vegetable Oils and Margarine

Margarine is a butter substitute made out of vegetable oils, which on their own are healthy but when hydrogenated to turn them solid, cause the oils to become trans-fats. When consumed, trans-fats thicken the blood, which forces the heart to work harder to pump it through our vessels, this in turn, raises blood pressure.

The fat content in our bodies are made up of 97% saturated and mono saturated fats. The final 3% is polyunsaturated fat in the form of Omega 3 and Omega 6. The omega cells are used for repairing and rebuilding cells. Margarine intake creates an unhealthy Omega 3 and 6 fatty acid ratio, which unbalances these finely tuned fats and therefore, the normal functioning of our cells.

Sunflower oils and corn oils have been found to produce high levels of chemicals called Aldehydes when heated up, which have been linked to heart disease, cancer and dementia. On high temperature frying, these oils produce twenty times more aldehydes than flaxseed or rapeseed oil and butter.

Eating fats after or combined with eating carbohydrates is detrimental to fat loss because on eating carbs, insulin levels are raised. Eating fat on top simply makes the fat cells fill up faster.

Recommended Oils for High Temperature Frying

Rapeseed oil

Coconut oil

Flaxseed oil

Foods To Eat and Why

Couscous

This is made from semolina granules and derives from North Africa. It is wonderfully easy to prepare, – just add boiling water, steam and fluff with a fork – and incredibly low in fat. A standard serving of couscous is only 176 calories or 8% of a 2000 calorie a day diet. It is also high in protein, one serving accounting for 12% of your recommended daily intake and makes up 39% of your recommended daily carbohydrate intake of 130 grams. It is high in vitamins and minerals including selenium, which is a powerful antioxidant known to reduce the plaque on vein and artery walls and prevent cancer. It reduces high blood pressure and keeps our fluids balanced due to its high potassium content.

It aids in fat loss, as it is a fiber rich food, which means it helps in the proper digestion of food and the general health and well being of the gastrointestinal system.

Rice

Rice has the ability to provide instant energy due to being abundant in carbohydrates. It stabilizes blood sugar levels and is a good source of the vitamin B1, which maintains a healthy nervous system and good cardiovascular function. There are 40,000 varieties of rice across the world, the main categories being wholegrain and white rice. Wholegrain rice, due to remaining largely unprocessed is high in nutrients.

Rice is low in fat, cholesterol and sodium and has

been proven to aid in weight loss.

Potatoes

Eaten plain, potatoes are fat free, rich in nutrients and low in calories. One potato is 110 calories containing 620 grams of potassium and 45% of your recommended daily intake of Vitamin C. There is no fat, sodium or cholesterol in a potato. Potatoes are what are known as a satiating vegetable in that one portion of potatoes, keeps you feeling full for an extended period of time. They are also nutrient dense for the amount of calories they hold.

There is often the assumption that potatoes are fattening, this is because they are rarely consumed in their basic form. Most potatoes that we know today come as French fries or roasted, sautéed and mashed.

Hummus

Hummus is made from chickpeas and is a popular North African staple. It is a protein rich food that balances blood sugar levels as it is slow to digest and not much needs to be consumed for the recipient to feel full. It contains iron and reduces cholesterol and is low in fat.

How To Make Hummus

Put the following into a blender and blend:

Ingredients

One can of chickpeas

One garlic clove

Three glugs of extra virgin olive oil

A sprinkle of cumin

A generous squeeze of lemon Juice

Method

Blend all the ingredients together until smooth.

Rainbow Veg

We all know eating five portions of fruit and vegetables a day (or is it ten now gotta keep up?) is essential for our health. It has been proven over and over again. Did you also know that different vegetables contain phytochemicals, which are naturally occurring plant chemicals, full of antioxidants, cancer reducing qualities, heart disease, eye problems, you name it. The way to get maximum phytochemicals from eating fruit and veg is to vary the colors of fruit and veg we eat. The more colors, the more phytochemicals, the more health benefits. Think Rainbow.

Red

Berries, tomatoes, peppers, red apples, rhubarb, cherries, and red grapes.

Red foods are rich in the antioxidant lycopene, which is what gives these foods their red color. Lycopene is an antioxidant shown to help protect against cancers.

Yellow/Orange

Oranges, pineapple, carrots, suede, sweet potato, sweet corn, peppers.

Yellow and orange foods are rich in vitamin A, which is essential for good vision and strong immune systems.

Green

Asparagus, cabbage, sprouts, broccoli, peas, lettuce, spinach, cucumber, pak choi, Chinese leaf – the list of greens is endless and the health benefits plentiful.

Good for the heart, for vision, for reducing risk of cancers – particularly breast and colon.

White

Onions, Jerusalem artichokes, turnips, parsnips, bananas.

Not really a rainbow color but white foods are rich in antioxidants, particularly garlic and onions. Also have been found to aid in reducing inflammation and allergies.

Eat a variety of these colors of vegetables and fruit to optimize the health benefits.

A typical daily diet for Phase One

Breakfast

100g of rice mixed with a boiled egg
Accompany this with a large glass of water

Mid Morning

Treat yourself to a medium baked potato with 30 grams of cooked chicken and a large glass of water
(If out working, this can be prepared the evening before and stored in a container.)

Lunch

100g of rice mixed with tuna and sweet corn and a large glass of water

(Again, if out working, this can be prepared the evening before and stored in a container.)

Mid afternoon

Take your pick of two pieces of fruit, ideally the same type; apples, pears, satsumas, oranges.

For tea

Mixed vegetables, around 100g ideally with 30g of fish – tuna, sardines, white fish – you choose.

Evening Meal

Round off the day with fruit and a large glass of water

PHASE TWO

The Incremental Reduction Phase

IN PHASE ONE, we discovered the health, vitality and fat reduction rewards that come about when we learn what foods are most beneficial to fat loss and health and also the effects of making small changes to our diet.

Phase Two is all about us taking control of our meals. By this we mean, becoming conscious of the amount of food we ingest and how this needs to be consistent with every meal. In order to do this, we need to be note takers taking notes of how much rice, protein and fiber is contained within each meal. This is much more important than counting our calories, which let's face it, can get complicated.

Phase Two is all about reducing what we ingest, little by little.

Reducing the amount eaten per meal and increasing the amount of meals per day, will cause the metabolism to ramp up its fat burning capacity as each smaller meal is processed and dealt with more efficiently than the previously larger meal portions described in Phase One.

Implementing Phase Two on Your Daily Mealtime

Part One

What is needed is a simple method for calculating the amount of each product by counting in tablespoons.

For example:

10 tablespoons of cooked rice,

3 tablespoons of chicken,

2 tablespoons of raw mixed colored vegetables

Take note of these amounts and become familiar with them.

Part Two

Now, using the daily diet in Phase One as an example, six meals over the course of the day, double these meals per day so that you have the same amount of food consumed but spread over 12 meals per day. Store these in meal containers so that they are always to hand.

It is important you maintain eating at regular times and do not skip meals in order to maximize the fat burning potency of this phase.

Part Three

Begin to reduce each meal you eat by one tablespoon of for example, rice. This means that of 12 total meals each meal would be reduced by one tablespoon giving you a total reduction over 12 meals of 12 tablespoons of rice.

Five Rules for Phase Two

1. Eat every two hours
2. Fill only two-thirds of your stomach
3. Always have a pre-prepared meal nearby
4. Fractionally reduce each meal portion
5. Introduce more mono meals (less varied food groups) in order to increase digestion and absorption of energy and nutrients

Repeat this with each meal component.

PHASE THREE

The Fine Tuning Phase

BY THIS PHASE OF THE FAT LOSS PROCESS, you will have achieved your ideal level of health vitality and fat reduction, but wait…. there's more!

Phase Three is about you making some slight changes that will help you to become the strongest version of yourself.

These tweaks are simple to undertake but will yield incredible rewards in terms of your body becoming even more healthy and your muscles defined as well as keeping your body burning fat, while quickly eliminating fat.

Negative Effects of Sodium

Firstly we need to work out the amount of sodium or salt that we consume daily. Knowing this is important because most of the population is far in excess of the RDA guidelines. This leads to issues within the body namely the amount of water and other fluids we unnecessarily hold on to.

Ingesting too much salt in your diet, leads to a condition known as edema, which comes about from water retention. The fluid accumulates in the subcutaneous layer beneath the skin lodging itself mainly in the abdomen region. Edema can lead to swollen ankles, legs, wrists and heart and kidney problems.

No amount of cardio or resistance training will remove fluid, as it is neither body fat nor muscle, however by reducing your salt/sodium intake, you will find your fluid levels will drop. Salt/sodium intake should be no more than 2000 milligrams or two grams per day.

If you cannot live without the seasoning, try *Cayenne Pepper* as a substitute. This is a great fat burning product due to its thermogenic effect, thermo meaning 'heat'. The thermogenic effect also facilitates the blood, stimulating the heart, lungs and circulatory system to eliminate waste materials. In addition it is packed full of vitamins and minerals.

Knowing your approximate daily intake of salt will enable you to gradually reduce this amount over the course of a week.

Ingesting Natural Substances for Optimizing Health

Apple Cider Vinegar

Vinegar lowers blood sugar levels, which gives you the feeling of being full. As a result, it reduces your calorie intake. Consuming a tablespoon (15ml) of vinegar a day has been proven to reduce belly fat and waist circumference.

Turmeric

This is the rootstalk of a tropical plant, part of the ginger family that turns curry, yellow. It is consumed in powder form and has been proven time and again to reduce the risk of cancer, liver damage, diabetes and Alzheimer's disease due to the compound curcumin, which is a powerful antioxidant.

One gram per day of turmeric extract is considered the best way of obtaining the health benefits of curcumin.

Root Ginger

This is very commonly used in alternative medicine. It can be consumed fresh, dried, powdered or as an oil. The main ingredient of the oil is gingerol, it is an antioxidant for use against cancers, heart disease and inflammations. The recommended dosage is two grams per day.

Sea Salt

Before you leap and shout with indignation, this is not the same as table salt mentioned above. Sea salt comes directly from the sea and does not go through any of the processing that interferes with its natural make up.

Believe it or not, sea salt has been shown to be an effective weight loss product. It helps the body create digestive juices that aid in digesting foods faster. It is also good for alkalizing the body and building a strong immune system. RDA is one teaspoon.

Chilli Powder

Makes sense right, something that heats you up, helps you burn fat. That will be the capsaicin, which is the chemical that adds the heat to chilli. Studies have found that one gram of cayenne pepper can work to reduce cravings for sweet, salty and fatty foods and increase energy expenditure.

Positive Effects of Distilled Water

Otherwise known as Still Water, this aids the flushing out of toxins alongside eliminating water retention. Keeping the body hydrated is essential to maintaining balance. Tea and coffee are best avoided in this phase as they act as diuretics causing the body to flush out water, which compromises the body's overall fluid content.

Coffee in particular, has a negative burnout effect on the adrenaline glands situated around the kidneys.

This can lead to mood disorders and reduce overall health. Herbal teas can be implemented as substitutes, which conversely hydrate the body with fluid as opposed to depleting it of water.

Top Tip

Eliminate stress. Working to eliminate stress within your life is crucial in both *Phases Two and Three* because of the gradual calorie deficit used to further reduce body fat levels. Stress namely stress hormones, released within the body can lead to water retention as well as issues relating to the cardiovascular system.

A certain level of daily stress is healthy and perfectly normal as it can push us beyond our perceived boundaries. Unnecessary or recurring stress, which serves no functional purpose, however, needs to be identified and remedied or avoided completely.

Sleep is key to reducing stress as it fosters health and restores equilibrium in the body. Many people are short-changing their efforts towards good health and fat reduction by simply not getting their minimum quota of undisturbed sleep. The average amount of 8 to 10 hours sleep per night is recommended.

Developing your own sleep ritual before you nod off can greatly improve the quality of rest.

The most common causes of a sleepless nights are social media platforms next to the bed, tea, coffee or adrenaline fuelled movies, which over stimulate the mind at the time of going to bed when we need to be relaxing our body and mind. Make a point of switching off your PC, laptop or handheld device two to three hours before bed and you will be amazed at the difference this makes toward a solid night's zzzzzzz.

Recap:

You are what you eat.

Eat well – live well. It is that simple. Eat unhealthily – crumble and rot.

Make small changes to your diet in order to increase its efficiency.

Juice every morning

Be conscious of the amount of food you ingest on a daily basis.

Ingest natural substances for optimal health.

Reduce stress.

Improve sleep.

Case Study

"Be the change that you wish to see in the world"
Mahatma Ghandi

Marie's Story

All her life, Marie now 34, suffered from gastro-intestinal issues; bloating, constipation and flatulence along with the skin condition, eczema. Growing up in a large family where her father had to work three jobs to bring food to the table and her mother was permanently time strapped due to tending to a stream of offspring, Marie bore her issues without ever being aware that what she was she was enduring was any different to anyone else.

The staple diet at home centered on 'foods that fill you up' namely, bread, pasta, potato, cereal and milk. There was never any 'fancy' food like pulses or vegetables extending beyond cabbages and carrots and even rice was considered 'exotic'.

Marie was never a child who 'enjoyed her food', her dad called her a 'fussy eater' and the times she complained of tummy aches (which was quite often) she was just laughed at and told to stop being 'soft' or to be 'grateful' for what she got. Having a petite frame, Marie was a slim child, made slimmer by her reluctance to eat.

As she entered adolescence and her early twenties, Marie started getting bad headaches and ulcers and for the first time, putting on weight. All this she put down to tiredness not that her life was particularly taxing but when aged 24, she was diagnosed with swollen joints, a combination of depression and inactivity, led her weight to almost double from 9 to 16 stone.

Going to work became problematic for Marie due to her office being on the top floor of a tower block where the lift was often out of order and walking up eight stories, was painful. She often called in sick, which in turn led to her needing doctor's notes.

The doctor prescribed her medication to relieve the swelling of her joints, known also to relax muscles and aid sleep but could not understand why Marie was not improving. When Marie told her she suffered from stomach pains, the doctor said it could be either heartburn and suggested a dose of antacids to neutralize the acids in her stomach or trapped wind telling Marie to avoid gassy foods such as cabbage, cauliflower, eggs, beans and sprouts.

Marie did not implement the doctor's advice because she did not believe deep down that they were the cause of her problems. Instead, she got it into her head that she might be suffering from something much more serious and became anxious desperately wanting someone who she could talk to about her concerns.

The anxiety led her to spend more time alone, which in turn gave her more opportunity to turn in on herself and fixate on her irrational worries. Rarely going out, she took to living off 'convenience' foods from the local store up the road. She became more bloated, the regularity of her headaches increased as did her weight and she was permanently tired.

At her local store one afternoon buying crisps and

ready-made pizza for lunch, Marie spotted a headline on a woman's health magazine saying *'Turn Up The Heat on Wheat'* The only reason it stood out to Marie was because beneath the word 'wheat' were the words, bloated, constipated and swollen joints.

Buying the magazine, Marie, through the course of reading the article, learnt more about food and diet than she had through a lifetime of eating. "It was speaking directly to me," Marie later said as she came to the realization that her diet was based almost 100% on wheat.

The article talked about the rapid increase in blood sugar levels that wheat produces; higher than the sugar rush from eating a bag of sweets. It also talked about wheat being addictive and stimulating appetite. Most importantly as far as Marie was concerned, however, was the link between wheat and obesity.

Interpretation

Having been brought up told to appreciate any food she could get as opposed to understanding the benefits of a balanced diet, it never crossed Marie's mind that her diet might be the cause of her problems. Good food to Marie was simply food that removed hunger pangs.

What she ate had forever been related to what she could afford. As a child meals were managed by her parents who would not tolerate any of the discomfort Marie was suffering because they were hard up. Food was hard to come by and they were too busy to give the time to Marie that she needed.

As an adult, managing her own meals, Marie had

rebelled against her mother's hard toil of cooking every dish from scratch and found the joys of ready meals and not just one ready meal per meal but several. Marie's stable diet growing up was largely wheat based and this was what she ate into adulthood because she knew no different.

The more wheat based products Marie ate, the more unwell she became as her body attempted to reject them and then adjust to the overeating of a grain that did not naturally digest in her system. By living off a fundamentally addictive food product, Marie never learned to pick up on the signals her body was putting out to inform her that she was full. Sometimes she found that even after eating a big bowl of pasta, she helped herself to more because she was craving the sugar rush.

This lead Marie not only to gain weight but also to suffer from the many health problems wheat can cause, especially if, like Marie, her body is wheat intolerant. It was wheat that was causing her swollen joints, her bloating, her constipation, anxiety and fatigue.

Outcome

Marie came to me by way of the article due to a mutual contact. She told me she wanted to lose weight, have more energy and live life as a 30-something should be living. On asking Marie what was a typical day's food intake, it became immediately apparent that she was eating a diet that was essentially poisoning her body. This was backed up by her obesity, the unhealthy color of her skin and the big bags under her eyes.

Marie's typical diet considered of Weetabix followed

by a jam sandwich for breakfast, wheat based ready meal for lunch, typically pizza or pasta and the same again in the evening. For snacks, she ate donuts, crisps or cupcakes.

I chatted to Marie about what she considered a healthy diet and her answer to me was simply, eating less. She did not understand food groups or balancing meals on a plate or the benefits of different colored foods, existing as she was on a largely brown and white diet.

There was a lot of work to do but Marie was very keen. It was as if after years of not listening to her body as it screamed out for help, she was suddenly waking up and wanting to make up for the decades of discomfort.

I informed Marie of the elimination diet, which in her case was centered largely on eliminating wheat. This, of course, concerned Marie who could not imagine what else she might eat if bread, pasta and cake were not permitted. We discussed together all of the other food groups such as the benefits of couscous, which she had never heard of, rice and potatoes and of how food on a plate should be made up of many colors, the main ingredients being vegetables.

Due to concerns that Marie by eradicating wheat might suddenly experience a sharp reduction in daily calories as she sought to understand appropriate replacements, I watched her closely. She was very quick to pick up on the benefits of other food groups although she was still reluctant to move away from purchasing ready meals and move onto preparing her own dishes. This, she told me, was a throwback to spending her childhood watching her mother toil over a hot stove. Together we discussed the joy of preparing meals from scratch, I made up a diet and recipe plan with quick to prepare dishes that were healthy and would 'fill her up', something still very important to Marie.

There was also a major focus on getting Marie to 'think ahead' and plan her daily meals. Her tendency was to buy food only when she was hungry. She got into the habit of preparing her evening meal prior to going to work in the morning investing in a slow cooker that ensured her meal put together first thing would be ready and steaming hot to look forward to when she got home. No toiling over a hot stove but healthy and low in fat.

I also encouraged Marie to invest in a juicer. This yielded the best results of all. Suddenly, after three decades of eating fruit only under duress, Marie was awash with all of the healthy vitamins a glass of fresh juice can provide. Her tendency to reach for a donut or jam sandwich was replaced with whooshing up apples, pears and bananas. Her sweet tooth was satisfied, she felt full and best of all, every day she lost weight.

Marie and I worked together for the best part of six months. Over this time, I watched her weight drop to the nine stone she naturally was. Her slim frame revealed itself along with a very well defined waist. She had boundless energy able to run up the steps to the top floor of her work without so much as a pause in breathing and everything about her shone.

She has managed to completely eliminate wheat from her diet. She is now mad about couscous, which by simply adding hot water, she finds more convenient that convenient foods, she is a major advocate of the humble potato, particularly baked, loves fruit and has found some of the most ingenious ways of ensuring she gets her five-a-day of veg.

I still keep in touch with Marie from time to time. She recently wrote an article for a health magazine about how eliminating wheat changed her life. All she needs to do now is work on her family and get them to swap the cupcakes for the couscous.

"Let me change the world first." Says Marie, "Before I attempt that gargantuan challenge."

CHAPTER FIVE

New Mountains To Climb

"Nothing can withstand the power of the human will if it is willing to stake its very existence to the extent of its purpose."

Benjamin Disraeli

CONGRATULATIONS!!!!

You have achieved your goal! You are now your ideal body weight and you look and feel fantastic.

You have undertaken an incredible feat and proven in the process that you can achieve anything you set your mind to.

So, go on, wallow in the glory of your success. Lap it up, Champ.

Done?

Good, so…. now for the rest of your life.

What's Next?

Once upon a time, the thought of taking part in a yoga class, jitsu or gymnastics would have been incomprehensible. What me? Gymnastics? Never!!

Am I right?

Well, times have changed buddy. Remember, you

look good, you feel good and you want to keep looking and feeling this way. You deserve it for all the hard work you've undertaken.

So, give your body the best in terms of physical efficiency and finesse. The more you do, the better you will feel mentally and physically.

Here are a few suggestions. Find what works best for you within the time frame you have and your lifestyle. Remember, though, a healthy body works in conjunction with a healthy mind. Feel good about yourself.

Yoga

Yoga focuses the mind, body and spirit into a state of one unit. Combining breathing exercises with physical exercise, it reinvigorates and energizes the body and mind to perform at its absolute best. The health benefits of yoga include: the strengthening of muscles, improved flexibility, perfecting the posture, increasing blood flow, decreasing blood pressure and building inner strength.

Brazilian Jiu-Jitsu

Brazilian Jiu-Jitsu is the king of all the martial arts. Pioneered by the Gracies, a prominent martial arts family from Brazil, it came to be an art in its own right, through the experimentation and adaptation of judo. By 'king of all the martial arts', we mean that it is the most effective and efficient way for self-defense in a fight/confrontation. This is not its only benefit though fear not, we are not sending you into battle. BJJ is different from other martial arts in that it focuses on grappling and ground fighting. Ninety per cent of fights go to the ground, yet most martial arts teach only standing techniques. BJJ also focuses on strategy as opposed to brute force so suits all shapes and sizes.

It teaches you body awareness and with awareness, strength and mobility soon follow. It toughens you physically and mentally and promotes persistence.

Practitioners of BJJ train to submission meaning when grappling is no longer an option, they submit to their opponent, usually when locked in a submission hold. Submission is communicated by way of a "Tap Out" whereby the opponent or the mat is tapped to signal defeat. It is this one salient characteristic of BJJ that sets it apart from almost all other martial arts. The goal being to dominate your opponent by first winning a submission.

Adult Gymnastics

Adult gymnastics courses teach you to perform in dynamic, adventurous ways. Adult classes are sometimes known as "Over The Hill" or "Adult Beginners" and based in Sports Centers. Sessions tend to begin with light cardio followed by stretching then on to some technical learning from forward rolls to cartwheel to, down the line, maybe backflips. Go for it.

Top Tip

If every step of the way, you find you are buffeted by misfortune, betrayal or lack of self belief, know that you are not alone, you are never alone. The universe that created you lives within you. You are it and it is you.

Listen to your inner compass. By letting it guide you, you are communing directly with the omnipotent universe that created the divine being that you are.

Recap:

You are the shape you want to be and you want to stay this shape so find a form of fitness that works for you.

A healthy body works in conjunction with a healthy mind.

Case Study

"Success is how high you bounce after you hit rock bottom"

General Paton

Ian's story

Ian was an active busy man with a job working night-clubs and bars, settling disputes and handling punters. A few years before, aged fourteen, he was diagnosed with a progressive eye condition known as RP, leading over time, to blindness. At first, he had no symptoms but as the years progressed, his vision deteriorated until his inability to see in the dark, made it too difficult for him to undertake his work duties.

Forced to quit his job, Ian found himself unemployed, inactive and drinking alone at night, sometimes getting through three bottles of wine in one sitting. He was isolated and deeply depressed. Old friends and relatives would visit him once in a while but for the most part, he was alone. Aware that he was no longer the man he had once been, classed now as disabled, Ian fell into despair.

A naturally private person, Ian did not share his inner turmoil and distress with his family or occasionally visiting friends, as he did not want to push them further away. He kept it bottled up binging on alcohol and processed food. Having always been in good shape, six foot tall and a pretty muscular 220lbs to 308lbs, his weight began to increase until his clothes no longer fitted him bar a few items, which would get worn and washed and worn again the next day.

He fell deeper into alcoholism and overeating to regulate his fluctuating mood.

Drunk and emotional one evening Ian was arrested by the police and the decision was made for him to be sent for psychiatric assessment.

Several weeks were spent in a secure unit as Ian was assessed. It was decided release would be permitted if Ian agreed to fortnightly injections with the purpose of regulating his mood. The injections were mandatory. Any refusal on Ian's part would result in police intervention.

Ian had hit rock bottom and was no longer the decision maker within his own life. He found this soul destroying and he was permanently in a state of fluctuating disbelief. After five years of mandatory injections, the decision was made to take Ian off the medication, by which time he neither cared one way or the other.

Interpretation

Instead of readjusting to his 'new life' as registered blind, Ian instead, gave into it and let the 'disability' take over. He considered himself a 'victim' and allowed others to see him as such until his self esteem was at rock bottom. He believed he had no power or control over his own life, a feeling further enforced by being on the mandatory medication.

Outcome

Free of the medication, Ian realized he had the chance to take back control, which he did by attempting to get his body into some sort of acceptable shape. Recalling his first workout, Ian remembers it consisting of ten squats alongside five pushups. With each exercise, his knees and elbows creaked. The repetitions were slow and labored and pathetic. He was exhausted. It felt like he had undertaken the most difficult workout ever performed. Years of inactivity and poor nutrition had taken their toll. The easy path here was to quit. Instead, though, he recorded the repetitions in his smart device.

In the following weeks and months, he began researching nutrition and exercise and motivational tools and through a process of experimentation and note taking, began to make progress. If he tried something and it yielded little or no result he discarded it and moved onto the next activity on his list.

In the end, he had built up what he considered to be the best, quickest and most efficient tools for sustained, healthy fat loss. Using the tools he quickly went down to 220lbs of lean body weight. The experimentation period was over and the tools he had assembled, worked better and more quickly than anything else he had experienced.

The pride he felt was enormous. He had persevered in the face of all odds and the fruits of his labor lay in the quality of his appearance and defined physique.

People began to compliment Ian as well as ask questions about what they could do to achieve the same results. He obliged by giving them exercises to try out to lose body fat. They came back to him explaining how well it had worked and thanking him. This praise boosted Ian further towards helping others until he eventually decided he would write a book containing everything he had learned on his journey.

The book became an over night bestseller and you are reading it now.

I am Ian, author of this book.

Thank you so much for purchasing my book. It has been a fantastic journey of discovery and an absolute honor to help you on your own personal journey.

Remember you can achieve and accomplish anything you set your mind to.

The sky is the limit. All you need do is identify your goal and Go!

www.ingramcontent.com/pod-product-compliance
Lightning Source LLC
Chambersburg PA
CBHW070251290326
41930CB00041B/2454

* 9 7 8 1 9 9 9 7 9 8 4 2 0 *